BUSINESS BEST-PRACTICES FOR SUCCESS IN MEDICARE'S VALUE-BASED HEALTH CARE PROGRAM

Nicole B. Dhanraj, Ph.D.

COPYRIGHT, 2017©

Business Best-Practices for Success in Medicare's Value-Based Health Care Program

By

Nicole B. Dhanraj, Ph.D.

This research study was completed as partial fulfillment of the requirements for the degree of

Doctor of Philosophy

on

Capella University, August 2013

Approved by:

Suzanne Richins, D.H.A., Faculty Mentor and Chair
Margaret Eggleston, Ph.D., Committee Member
Stuart Gold, Ph.D., Committee Member
Barbara Butts Williams, Ph.D., Dean,
School of Business and Technology

Abstract

Within the health-care industry, numerous quality improvement strategies exist to promote a more efficient and effective system. Despite such strategies, the health-care system is yet to experience sustained quality improvement. Value-based health care is a pecuniary strategy established by the Center of Medicare and Medicaid Services to achieve sustained improvement, both in the delivery of care and in clinical outcomes.

With a value-based strategy, Medicare provided only clinical process measures as a guideline for organizations in delivering higher quality. This strategy situation may create difficulties for organizations in selecting the most suitable business strategies that maintain a quality-financial balance. Leaders are left to guess at business strategies that are most optimal for success in the program, as well as for the organization's financial sustainability.

Sustained improvement in the health-care industry can be accelerated when leaders are knowledgeable on appropriate strategies important to increasing the value and quality of care, while reducing waste. This exploratory qualitative study used the Malcolm Baldrige Criteria for Performance Excellence as a quality improvement tool for exploring the business strategies can promote clinical and financial success for organizations participating in Medicare's value-based program.

The findings derived from responses to semi-structured interviews of 21 health-care, leader-participants were triangulated with publicly available, published documents from health-care organizations. Recommended future research includes identification of strategies specific to non-profit, for-profit, and government owned health-care organizations.

Dedications and Acknowledgement

My research study is dedicated to my husband, parents, grandparents, and dearest friends. To my incredible soul mate, Elvis Dhanraj, the core of my being; I cannot thank you enough for your continued loving support. You have been my cheerleader in this journey. You have nurtured me and blessed me with your words of love. You have and will always continue to provide support for my dreams no matter how grandiose. Your love is breathtakingly pure and wider than the ocean. Shakespeare said, "The course of true love never did run smooth," but he never met a couple like us! I love you, MBZT!

To my mother, Molly Joseph, you have always encouraged me reach beyond the stars. Your mantra, 'its sockeye' made me never doubt my abilities. I was always willing to try, especially when you were my biggest cheerleader. Your desire for me to always be 'numero uno' provided me the encouragement to take on this sacred journey. You were always there to help me balance work, school, and family – despite worrying about me constantly being on the go. I love you endlessly!

In loving memory of my father, Cyril Vernon Joseph; you instilled in me the importance of education and always reiterated 'knowledge is power.' You always expected beyond the best from me and I know you would be proud of this ostentatious accomplishment. Your stories and lessons will always be cherished in my heart.

To my children, Avinash, Ameerah, and Ariana, who never complained about the countless hours I spent in the office; I love you all to the moon and back! You provided special support, spending time with me in the office, or just snuggling next to me while writing. Thank you for your patience and understanding!

Heartfelt thanks to my grandfather, Ramnarine Mahadeo (Nana), who made me thirsty for learning. You never doubted your grandchildren's abilities, showed excitement at our accomplishments, and kept us in your prayers. I know you are beaming with pride.

In loving memory of my grandmother, Sookdaye Mahadeo; I wish you could have seen this accomplishment. I know you too would be overjoyed.

To my closest friends, Jack McDaniel, Mark Lockwood, and Parsuram 'Ram' Ramkisson; a very special thank you for your unending support and belief in me, especially when I doubted myself. You kept me grounded and ensured I smelled the roses; I am honored to be called your friend. The journey to complete this dissertation could not have been done without the support of many other colleagues, family, and friends. Special thanks go to all those who have made their mark in my life. Thank you for your faith in me and the inspiration to be the best. It is God's will for me to be abundantly blessed!

Dr. Suzanne Richins, your expertise helped me stay focused and motivated to the end. Thank you for your commitment and dedication; without you, this success would be impossible. To my mentors, Dr. Eggleston and Dr. Gold, thank you for your feedback, advice, and encouragement.

My Capella colleagues – Leslies Kayanan, Angela Mosby, Kathryn Meagher, Kim Vetter, Heidi Nguyen, and Patrick Davis; you all have cheered me on, provided an enormous amount of advice, picked me up when I was lost, and inspired me to finish this journey. I am eternally grateful for our discussions and continued faith that I can get it done.

To Jessica Sawyer, I have always admired your ability to stay focused and balanced in life. You provided great life lessons and dared me to believe in myself beyond my years and capabilities. You have inspired me never to underestimate my abilities.

To Sister Mary Olivia, my adopted mother; I am grateful you took me under your wings and nurtured me – both spiritually and academically. Your prayers, love, and support set the foundation for me to become the adult I am today.

To everyone else who has helped me through this journey and contributed to the accomplishment of this dream, I am forever indebted. Thank you all!

Nicole B. Dhanraj, Ph.D.

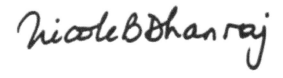

Table of Contents

List of Tables

List of Figures

Chapter 1

Introduction

In a seminal report prepared for the Institute of Medicine (IOM), Kohn, Corrigan, and Donaldson (2000) revealed the United States health-care system was in a poor and adverse state, and it continued to remain in this state (Wachter, 2010). Subsequently, the IOM recommended a comprehensive strategy for change. Government and quality agencies embarked upon change through a variety of improvement strategies.

Strategies included implementing regulations, adding new responsibilities for health-care professionals, education, and change initiatives in a variety of areas such as organizational processes (Sherwood, 2012). Efforts were successful and brought about short-term improvements (Repenning & Sternman, 2001). Despite these efforts, problems of inefficiencies, waste, unsafe practices, inequitable care, unnecessary volumes, and rising expenditure persisted (R. Bush, 2007; Wachter, 2004, 2010). These problems amounted to roughly 30% of health-care spending and translated to roughly $765M annually (Fineberg, 2012). It was evident the industry continued to lack sustained practices to promote cost-efficiency and high quality.

In 2013, strategies had not yielded sustainable improvements as the nation continued to experience poor service and poor outcomes with escalating costs. For the resources consumed in health care, outcomes were unsatisfactory and the value of service did not commensurate with dollars spent. A 2012 estimate by the Centers for Disease Control and Prevention (CDC) reported 99,000 deaths because of health-care associated infections and more than 700,000 injuries and deaths from adverse medication reactions (U.S. Department of Health and Human Services, 2013). Some of the patients who developed hospital acquired infections and other medical errors often needed additional services to treat the outcomes of these issues. In 2011, an estimated $2.7T (USD) was spent in health care (Hartman, Martin, Benson, & Catlin, 2013). This increase in spending was an almost 4% increase from 2010. In 2011, costs were roughly 18% of the gross domestic product (GDP), with a 4% increase from 2000. This was projected to increase to 21% by 2023 (Peterson & Burton, 2011; Schoen, 2013). Expenditures and resources dedicated to health care may have been warranted, if there were excellent outcomes in clinical care.

Resources and expenditures in the health-care industry are not dedicated to bringing about excellent outcomes for patients. Berwick and Hackbarth (2012) and Kumar, Ghildayal, and Shah (2011) suggested much of the increase in health-care spending was from unnecessary waste. These authors identified waste resulting in non-adoption of best-care practices, fragmented care, overtreatment, misguided or inefficient rules, pricing failures, and fraud. In addition to the lack of return on investment (ROI; money spent), excessive resources devoted to health care alone choked investments in other areas of the country such as education, public safety, and community development programs (Muenning & Glied, 2010). Investments in these noted areas may have provided additional benefits to patients instead of the patients needing further medical care.

Compared to other countries, the United States' health-care costs are highest in comparison. The United States did not have more efficient or better care than other countries, especially since the life expectancy of patients was no longer compared to other countries (IOM, 2012). The United States had the third highest death rate from medical errors. Infant mortality and life expectancy was no better than other countries that spend less on health care. Critics argue it was impossible to compare countries, as metrics of reporting may be different or their health-care system may have varied characteristics; as such, evidence will vary according to the context. Muenning and Glied (2010) conducted a study to determine if mortality rates and life expectancy were a result of an inefficient and defective system or merely because of poor personal health habits. The researchers found the United States continued to under-perform in comparison to other countries within aspects of similar behavioral health habits; in some instances, behavioral habits were improved (greater decline in smoking habits or slow growth of obesity) compared to the other countries. Muenning and Glied reported that for 30 years, the United States consistently fell behind other nations with respect to the 15-year survival of both genders in the age group between 45 and 65. Therefore, Muenning and Glied offered the poor performance of the United States' health-care system was not because of behavioral habits, but because of the nature of the health care and/or medical-related system.

In relation to expenditures, quality and outcomes in the United States were inversely proportional compared to other countries. Squire (2012) found the United States' health care quality was not superior compared to those countries spending considerably less. Squire said, in comparison to the United States health-care system, the Japanese system contained similar features such as advanced technology, fee for service payment, and unrestricted access to care. Japan's health care expenditure grew only 2% in the past 30 years compared to a growth of 8% in the United States. Although Squire (2012), Kumar et al. (2011), and Muenning and Guild (2010) implied a fragmented and inefficient health-care system accounted for the poor outcomes, no details on the variance of the internal processes of the countries compared were provided. Squire (2012) noted if the United States spent the same amount as Japan, the United States could recognize a potential savings of $1.25 trillion dollars. Neither Squire nor other researchers offered a comparison of clinical or business processes. Squire echoed appeals by the United States government and other reporting agencies for a need for more transparency and standardization to promote efficient, equitable, and higher quality of care.

As health-care technology continued to soar, it was even more imperative leaders undertook movements to improve quality of care, increase safety, and reduce unnecessary costs. Chassin and Loeb (2011) suggested a main reason for the poor quality in health care was the continual introduction of new equipment, medication, and procedures that increased the complexity of delivering health care – safe, effective, and valuable. The United States would not be able to sustain health-care spending as it was projected to continue. For the dollars spent, there were no impressive returns, especially in terms of increasing the value of care delivered or improving the quality of life for patients (Peterson & Burton, 2011; Schoen, 2013). As a result, the entire health-care system needed a critical evaluation in both its systematic and clinical processes (Muenning & Glied, 2010; Squires, 2012; U.S. Department of Health and Human Services, 2010, 2013). Such an evaluation could contain costs into a more sustainable range (Berwick & Hackbarth, 2012). Chassin and Loeb (2011) suggested it was necessary to look at organizations outside the health-care industry to gain a better picture of how best to make improvements and to stabilize health costs, so it properly matches GDP growth.

Although the opportunities to improve were enormous, a key lesson recognized from organizations outside the health-care industry was to have a high degree of reliability and accountability in organizational processes. This focus resonated with Kohn et al.'s 2001 report for the IOM, which highlighted the payment structure for health-care services lacking accountability for the value of services provided. Reimbursement methods reinforced improper organizational practices and processes by paying according to volume and complexity, rather than based on performance or value. The report implied the unified thinking within health-care organizations was 'more medical care' meant 'better quality care'; therefore, spending less on health-care services meant reduced quality and poor outcomes.

Although there was literature on quality improvement practices, a reason offered for the continued experience of waste and poor quality was organizations always received payments – regardless of the quality of service provided or outcomes. There was no motivation or incentive to perform better (Robinson, 2001). Repenning and Sterman (2001) attributed this lack of motivation from the unsupportive cultural mindset to quality improvement and structure of the organization. Traditionally, Centers for Medicare and Medicaid Services (Medicare) paid for health care service regardless of the quality or costs of services members received. Medicare's spending jumped 14 times from 1980 to 2010. Resources devoted to health care, as of 2010, were $522 billion, which was 45% of the national expenditure (H. Bush, 2012). This guaranteed reimbursement resulted in inefficient use of resources, perpetuated substandard care, and in some cases, rewarded poor quality of care through reimbursement of additional services that, perhaps, were unnecessary. Officials within Medicare recognized the lack of reliability in health care and promised its beneficiaries to increase accountability, improve the quality of care, and rein in costs to maximize the potential of its programs and, in turn, the value to its customers (Fenter & Lewis, 2008). Subsequently, Medicare officials implemented a strategy that paid hospitals for quality and performance in the care they delivered.

To address the deficiency in the fee-for-service payment system, the IOM committee offered a pay-for performance plan (P4P) for Medicare to implement a plan that "would address current problems and stimulate complementary quality improvement strategies" (Kohn et al., 2001, p. 5). The Institute made two suggestions: promote the quality of care envisioned within the health-care industry and provide payment methods that encouraged a redesign of structures and processes within organizations. The report continued, noting that although it was uncertain about the size of incentive needed to bring about significant change, it was important to address the deficiency of the payment system. This report was part of a series of IOM reports published in its efforts to accelerate quality improvement and to reduce waste within the healthcare industry.

In 2010, the need to fix the US health care crisis arose because of the increasing spending burden on the already failing economy. The Obama administration implemented the Affordable Care Act in 2010 with the assertion the health-care system will improve and therefore function in a more efficient and effective capacity (Patient Protection and Affordable Care Act, 2010). The purpose of implementation of the Affordable Care Act was to make health care affordable to all, increase access to care, hold insurance and health-care organizations accountable for their actions, ensure transparency in the quality of services and improve their practices, not only the quality in services delivered, but the outcomes of care patients received. A National Strategy for Quality Improvement in Health Care was developed. These goals aligned with the IOM's aims of a better health-care system, which meant organizations promised delivery of improved quality of care, reduced costs, and were supportive of the appropriate interventions (U.S. Department of Health and Human Services, 2013). These initiatives helped spur new efforts for quality improvement in health care.

The Affordable Care Act spurred reform in one of the nation's largest payers of medical services, Medicare. Public purchasers of health care no longer just paid for services as it did previously (Pettypiece &

Armour, 2013). Instead, Medicare representatives began to scrutinize the value of every dollar spent in relation to clinical outcomes. In 2013, Medicare officials attempted to reduce excessive costs through evaluating, scrutinizing, and increasing the expectations of the value of care received for dollars spent. To improve the value of care received per health-care dollars spent, Medicare officials said they intended to hold health-care organizations accountable for quality of care provided and expected these organizations to increase operating efficiency and reduce long-term expenses. In 2009, Medicare officials defined this approach as value-based purchasing. Under the bonus plan, Medicare intended to withhold 1% of payments based on the organization's scores in clinical-related measures. By 2017, Medicare officials' intentions were to withhold up 2% of payments (Pettypiece & Armour, 2013). By 2013, the officials identified areas where organizations could have improved their procedures.

The concept of value-based health care is to change organizational behavior and practices and emphasize a value-based approach. A reimbursement strategy provided incentives to encourage quality improvement in care. This, in turn, leads to higher performance with improved outcomes and lower utilization costs (Fenter & Lewis, 2008). Leaders were encouraged to deliver a higher quality of care and reduce unnecessary costs. Medicare, hospitals, states, and others have been experimenting quietly since 2007 to evaluate and improve the quality of clinical outcomes and control the unnecessary costs for their beneficiaries. Medicare used a phased approach to introduce the program, so lessons learned could help with subsequent changes and redevelopment of models that met their goals (Cromwell, Trisolini, Pope, Mitchell, & Greenwald, 2011). These efforts focused on clinical measures and health-care outcomes.

Although organizations continued to improve in their workplace and health care processes to meet the goals of value-based health care, evidence-based research focused more on clinical initiatives and less on business strategies that were the foundation of ensuring organizational sustainability (H. Bush, 2012). Such business strategies may have been beneficial to the success of value-based health care. Chassin and Loeb (2011) suggested, "Leadership commitment, full implementation of a safety culture and thorough adoption of robust process improvement tools, and methods together is the pathway most likely to lead to success" (p. 568). The problem was the focus of the efforts was mainly on improving the quality, efficiency, and outcomes of clinical practices. Of the literature reviewed, there was no other evidence of business strategies that could help organizations' leaders achieve success in their organization's clinical goals resulting in earning the organization's maximum reimbursement.

Redefining Health Care

The initial suggestion to remedy the deficiencies within the health-care system stemmed from IOM's reports, *To Err is Human: Building a Safer Health System* (Kohn et al., 2000) and *Crossing the Quality Chasm: A New Health System for the 21st Century* (Kohn et al., 2001). These reports indicated errors resulted from inefficient, ineffective, and variable processes within the system. These reports emphasized improvements in health-care delivery should have six goals: safety, effectiveness, patient-centric, timely, equitable, and efficient for all persons (IOM, 2001). The reports urgently prompted health-care leaders to act, which some did; more so, what resulted was more a competitive reaction or regulatory compliance than of moral obligation or encouragement to fix the system.

Background of the Study

Increased spending placed a tremendous burden on the economy, especially resulting from the recession (circa late 2007 to 2010). As a result, the government increased its focus on health-care spending and quality improvement in the industry (U.S. Department of Health and Human Services, 2010). Since 2005, the attempt at cost containment achieved minimal long-term effect, thereby prompting several proposals to encourage reform (Chassin,

Loeb, Schmaltz, & Wachter, 2010). As of 2012, Medicare officials hoped to reduce costs and improve quality by financially rewarding organizations based on clinical outcomes and patient feedback of services provided (CMS, 2012). Medicare officials evaluated services based on value of care provided as opposed to volume, as previously relied on by most organizations. As of 2014, regardless of whether health-care organizations were prepared, Medicare was to fully implement the program (CMS, 2012). This effort was a key endeavor to promote a safer and higher quality of care at reduced costs.

Several attempts at health-care reform had occurred beginning with multiple-government reform laws from President Clinton's managed care approach in the 1990s, which called for universal coverage and controlled costs, to the Deficit Reduction Act of 2005, which made significant changes to Medicaid. Such reforms were more concerned with compliance of guidelines for organizations to remain competitive and decrease costs to help ease the financial burden (U.S. Department of Health and Human Services, 2012). Other efforts included integrative strategies in 2005 and 2007 by the Commonwealth Fund, and the Engelberg Center for Health-Care Reform, as well as the IOM Roundtable on Value and Science-Driven Health Care in 2006. The main ideas of the strategies were to "turn a behemoth health care complex into a more streamlined health system that delivers greater value for the money" (Fineberg, 2012, p. 1022). In the years 1999-2009, quality improvement efforts in health-care industry included more robust standards of accreditation, improved use of information technology, payment penalties, better use of quality metrics, and increased emphasis on error-reporting (Chassin et al., 2010; "Why not the best?" 2011). However, despite these efforts and scattered pockets of excellence, the health-care industry has not consistently maintained continued optimum levels of safety and quality (Chassin & Loeb, 2011). A framework to improve the system holistically, rather than in specific areas, was deficient.

The fragmented system lacks the proper framework to ensure a healthier competition, that did not come at the expense of patients, through disparities in cost and care. Fragmentation, argued Muenning and Glied (2010), led to increased medical errors because of poor communication amongst the multiple providers involved in patient care and because of the conflicting instructions for patients from these different providers. Fragmentation within the system was also responsible for excessive administrative costs, as organizations must spend a great deal of time monitoring and complying with regulations and implementing strategies to deal with possible poor outcomes (Schoen, 2013). A guideline of business strategies to help organizations transition from the traditional fee-for-service to fee-for-performance would have helped facilitate success.

Statement of the Problem

The problem in Medicare's value-based reimbursement program was a lack of knowledge of business strategies existing to promote achievement of clinical-quality measure outcomes, increased value of care delivered, and maximum reimbursement for services provided. A lack of knowledge existed on how health-care leaders could achieve a balance between improvement of quality outcomes and financial sustainability.

Purpose of the Study

The purpose of this exploratory case study was to fill the gap of knowledge by exploring the business practices health-care leaders used successfully to support improvement in the leader's respective organizations in the value of care delivered for patients, achievement of clinical quality measures, and ultimately to receive maximum reimbursement for services provided. A secondary purpose of the study was to explore how leaders achieved a balance between quality improvement and financial sustainability. The exploratory research study used the Malcolm Baldrige Criteria as a tool to identify practices participants use to improve quality in their organizational processes and the value of care delivered to patients. The flexible and naturalistic design of this exploratory study allowed the researcher to explore the phenomenon of value-based health care while using participants' responses and content of the public documents as the units of analysis. This study used inductive and content analysis on data collected from responses of 21 participants to a semi-structured interview questionnaire and 24 random public organizational documents. This insight allowed identification of themes within the Malcolm Baldrige Criteria to determine practices that facilitated success in value-based, health care in this case study.

Rationale

Since implementation of the value-based concept, the focus has been primarily on improving the quality and outcomes of clinical practices, such as fibrinolytic therapy received within 30 minutes of hospital arrival, prophylactic antibiotic received within one hour prior to surgical incision, readmissions for certain medical conditions such as acute myocardial infarction heart failure and pneumonia within 30 days of discharge (CMS, 2011). The leadership within Medicare provided organizations with standards expected in clinical outcomes to achieve maximum reimbursement. Organizations needed to identify, through trial and error, the best practices that achieved the quality of care expected, practices that ensured maximum reimbursement, and therefore organizational financial sustainability. The problem faced by health-care organizations was the method by which health-care organizations could deliver a high quality of care with the threat of reduced reimbursement, but also be able to sustain those efforts to deliver the care expected. There was no evidence, at the time of this study's publication, that identified an associated framework of organization for implementation as a guide to ensure success.

An understanding of business practices that leads to improved outcomes could avoid a trial-and-error approach. Organizational leaders cannot afford to guess what will work. Hospital leadership needs to choose rationally, for a given course of action, to ensure benefits associated with the action(s) did not exceed costs. Organizational leadership needs to maintain the balance between quality health care and the institution's financial goals, requiring an assessment of the benefits of the chosen actions based on preferences. It is the underlying strategic processes that represented the core functioning of the organization and a lack of understanding that could result in problems (Skrinjar, Bosilj-Vukšic, & Indihar-Štemberger, 2001). Lack of knowledge of the critical factors that should encourage success in value-based, health care was an impediment to surpassing expected performance outcomes, and ultimately financial viability.

Although larger and more financially stable organizations could have worked on a trial-and-error basis to determine more valuable business strategies, smaller organizations did not have such an advantage. This disadvantage potentially could have led to increased and unnecessary costs, poor use of resources, financial demise, propagation of sub-optimal, health care, and ultimately a broken health-care system. From the literature review, past research focused on quality improvement in terms of identifying quality indicators, methods to reduce medical errors, explanatory cause and effect concepts, and methods to measure performance. Leadership in organizations relied on experience to steer the organization in a successful direction.

Currently, evidence was devoted to examining the best practices, which organizations could use to foster success in value-based purchasing ... to increase the value of care, while reducing costs ... was lacking. Therefore, it was important that research was conducted to determine evidence-based practices to transform healthcare, so leaders could avoid waste and inefficiency.

Leaders should establish evidence-based practices, choose processes to enable projected outcomes, and strive for holistic and positive outcomes for the business (Montgomery, 2010). Present research attempted to fill the literature gap by providing leaders with a guideline of business strategies that influences strategic decisions, which ultimately will accelerate success in use of a value-based, care initiative.

Research Questions

Research questions established the foundation and methodology for the research project. The research questions guided data collection to obtain an understanding of participants' experience with the strategies that promoted improvement in efficiency, delivery of a higher quality of care, and ensuring full reimbursement for services provided. The research questions in this study were comprised of one main question and one sub-question:

1. What are the best business strategies health-care leaders could use to increase the value of care delivered for success in Medicare's value-based health care program?

   a. How do leaders achieve a balance between increasing the value of care delivered, and sustainment of their organization's financial growth?

Significance of the Study

Although the goals of clinical value-based health care are clear, as presented by Medicare, there may be difficulty in implementing processes to achieve the goals for a variety of reasons. In the literature reviewed, evidence suggested a strategy is lacking to fulfill the performance measures of value-based, health care. AHRQ reported, "Knowing where to focus efforts improves the efficiency of interventions" (AHRQ, 2011 p. 1). The study's intent was to qualitatively explore business best practices that organizations could employ to ensure those business practices are effective, efficient, produce high quality services; to identify business practices to ensure care delivery was rooted in value. The measures Medicare officials identified helped determine if provided care was good or bad. A focus solely on measures and outcomes cannot assess underlying causes that affect variations and outcomes in quality. Montgomery (2010) stated that quality strategic planning is the foundation of success; without it, organizations can experience further waste in resources, defects in designs, and customer dissatisfaction. A structured strategic approach to quality is an integral part in quality improvement.

This research study's findings could have significant value for organizations participating in Medicare's value-based health care. This research study's findings could serve as a guideline for organizations to aid the health-care organizations in meeting the expectations of Medicare and helping sustain the organization financially, while delivering high-quality patient care. A focus on clinical outcomes and improving clinical initiatives was a one-sided improvement effort and did not help organizations prepare to deliver greater value from their investments. Jacob, Madu, and Tang (2012) stated, "to excel as an organization, much more than quality is needed" (p. 234). It was of value for organizations to have evidence-based data of effective business strategies that worked best to ensure efficiency, accountability, and – ultimately – their own success. The results of this research study would add to the literature by Medicare presented organizations with clinical outcomes expected for attainment of a higher standard of quality in health care. Leadership within Medicare emphasized value rather than volume for reimbursement purposes.

Value-based health care is the health care of the future, especially as Medicare was one of the largest payers of health-care services; commercial payers often followed Medicare's lead. To sustain financial and long-term growth, it was imperative for health-care leaders in medical and health-care organizations, even those not yet participating in Medicare's value-based program, to understand the business strategies important for implementation and execution of business processes to achieve national goals of quality health care. Medicare officials are trying to improve quality, efficiency, and accountability within the health-care system via a transformation of the payment structure to a system that rewards value rather than volume. Continued research in this area will foster organizational success and be advantageous to business' productivity and profit margins. When costs and quality concerns are aligned, value-based care could be accelerated, thus reforming health care to achieving national quality goals in the United States.

Time was critical in determining best business strategies that supported value-based health care. According to data from Medicare, about 50% of health-care organizations participated in the program by 2014. By January 2016, the pay-for-performance program was mandatory for psychiatric hospitals, long-term care, and hospice hospitals, as well as rehabilitation hospitals (CMS, 2011). This change meant, between 2014 and 2017, organizational leaders needed to understand the influence between business strategies and achieving quality levels desired, reducing costs, and increasing efficiency in practices and processes.

Organizations needed to choose appropriate practices to maintain value-based health care, especially as components direct influences on subsequent practices. This study was imperative for continued operational and financial sustenance of health-care organizations, so institutions could use resources appropriately to reduce waste, increase value of services, and deliver the quality of health care as the system intended.

In 2006, Epstein alluded that eventually business measures should be tied to efficiency measures, but advised that doing so would be challenging. The literature review did not identify any research that addressed best practices in Medicare's value-based concept. It was significant to identify research to report the business practices needed to provide a sense of direction as organizations transition to system of value-based health care.

The outcomes of this research study could fill the gap of a lack of knowledge of the business strategies that promoted success in Medicare's value-based health care program. These were the areas where the goals of value-based care, clinical outcomes – as prescribed by CMS – and organizational excellence intersected (see Figure 1). The outcomes of this study could serve as a guide for health-care organizations to utilize business strategies in categories of leadership, organization strategy, and performance measures. The outcomes should aid leaders in providing the quality of care expected for 100% reimbursement by Medicare, and to fulfill the expectations of the organization's patients. This research study could also encourage organizational leaders to improve business and performance improvement dashboards, and therefore be more accountable for clinical outcomes. The research study could help these health-care organizations maintain or achieve the institution's quality-financial alignment and success in Medicare's value-based program.

Goals of Value-Based Care

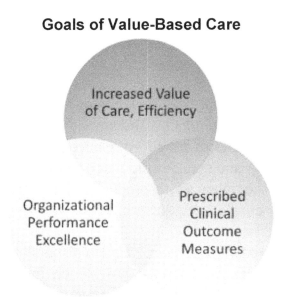

Figure 1 - Gap of Knowledge

Definition of Terms

Use of terminology for this study follows:

Best practices are a technique established by means of experience and research, and has proven to give a desired outcome. The practices consistently produce positive outcomes with replication (Gamm, Hutchison, Dabney, & Dorsey, 2003).

Effective: For the purpose of this study, effective refers to the delivery of a satisfactory and high quality output.

Efficient: For the purpose of this study, efficient refers to achieving results without wasting time, effort, or resources.

Health care expenditures as a proportion of gross domestic product: "The amount of health care goods and services produced relative to the amount of all goods and services produced represents the share of the nation's total production that is attributed to health care" (CMS, 2011, p. 18).

Health disparities: "Health disparities are differences in the incidence, prevalence, mortality, and burden of diseases and other adverse health conditions that exist among specific population groups in the United States" (National Institute of Health, 1999, p. 3).

Malcolm Baldrige Criteria for Performance Excellence are a set of guidelines composed of seven categories of indicators that address components of business excellence and improvement in organizations. The categories are "leadership, strategic planning, customer/ market focus, workforce focus, operation focus, measurement, analysis, and knowledge, and results" (National Institute of Standards and Technology [NIST], 2013, p. iii).

Quality is the attributes that makes a product or service superior and results from performance excellence by the organization (American Society for Quality, 2013).

Quality Improvement consist of the actions for improving the processes and outcomes of health care, including "increasing value; improving responsiveness to customers and consumers; improving outcomes in the areas of safety, effectiveness, timeliness, patient centeredness, equity, and efficiency; reducing variation in outcomes; and increasing organizational adoption and implementation of continuous improvement methods in ongoing operations" (Alexander & Herald, 2009, p. 240).

Value is defined as "patient health outcomes achieved relative to the costs of care" (Porter, 2010, p. 2478).

Assumptions and Limitations

Assumptions

The assumptions for this study are as follows:

1. The topic of value-based health care was relatively new, so it was assumed the proposed research would be of benefit to facilities who have not yet implemented this approach.
2. It was assumed the participants would be willing to share their best practices in attaining value-based health care and therefore offer full participation.

3. In addition, it was assumed the research would help those health-care organizations struggling to meeting the aims of this approach in addition to business goals, especially financial.
4. The research was conducted upholding ethical considerations for participants.
5. The research guidelines for a qualitative study were followed to ensure the study's validity and reliability.
6. It was assumed participants had ample experience in developing, implementing, and changing strategies to promote quality improvement.

Limitations

The limitations were as follows:

1. The method of inquiry chosen for this research limited the research. A quantitative study provides more objectivity and provides a larger number of participants, a qualitative case study was appropriate to discover experiences of strategies that fulfilled goals of value-based health care.
2. A qualitative methodology limited the study such that findings from qualitative studies could not be generalized beyond the participants of this research. Findings could ease the transition to value-based health care, especially for those not participating yet in the program or struggling to meet the institution's quality-financial alignment.

3. The researcher was the data collection instrument, thus there was the possibility of bias and personal influence existing that could result in data misinterpretation. The researcher attempted to limit bias by making notes and report any emotions or comments as they arose. Interviews were recorded to facilitate repeated listening or accuracy in reporting. The findings of this research study were reported as interpreted using critical thinking and reasoning. To minimize any misinterpretation of responses or published data, participants were presented with findings to ensure the essence of responses were captured accurately.

4. The study was inclusive of organizations across the United States. There may be additional factors such as geographic location, population, size, or ownership that could have influenced responses to interview questions, and as such may not have provided a consistent guideline to strategies that worked best in achieving the goals of value-based health care.

5. Research experience and research time constrained the researcher. The research was limited to available participants, as well as publicly available documents.

Theoretical Framework

After a review of the literature, no theoretical framework was found specific to business strategies of value-based health care. The theoretical framework rests in the theory of total quality management. Quality pioneers such as Deming, Juran, Shewhart, and Crobsy were key contributors to quality improvement concepts.

The underlying principles of this theory reflected these pioneers' philosophy on elements of quality. The Total Quality Management (TQM) theory serves as the foundation to other variants of the model (Samson, & Terziovski, 1999). Key components of total quality management follow:

1. The consumer was the most important part of the organization; therefore, quality changes occur according to the needs of the customer.
2. Organizational leaders were the drivers of quality management.
3. Quality improvement focused on the preservation of the organization through integration of multiple business processes.
4. Issues of quality were systematic and involved processes – part of a product and service design.
5. Quality improvement was a continuous journey that drives organizations to meet changing expectations of customer and environment.
6. Data on how organizations are performing was critical to improvement.

7. Quality management should be the core of strategic planning.

Conceptual Framework

The study used the Malcolm Baldrige Criteria for Performance Excellence (MBCPE) as the conceptual framework to bridge the gap in knowledge of organizational strategies for performance excellence in value-based health care research. The Malcolm Baldrige National Quality Award (MBNQA) was established in 1987 to recognize organizations for their high quality and excellent performance (NIST, 2008). The Malcolm Baldrige Criteria has been used by various organizations as an appropriate, all-inclusive, quality-improvement tool to help organizations manage key business activities for success through continued organizational excellence and sustainability. Since 1987, the Baldrige criteria has provided a means for "promoting exemplary quality management practices" (Flynn & Saladin, 2001, p. 617).

The Malcolm Baldrige model was a catalyst to reshaping attitudes and behavior toward quality improvement and has been used by numerous organizations in various industries since inception. As shown in Figure 2 (following), the MBCPE criteria was a conceptual framework for operationalizing quality management in previous studies (Dellana & Hauser, 1999; Handfield & Ghosh, 1995); therefore, the criteria were a means for operationalizing value-based health care as an organizational strategy for improvement and excellence.

Pre-Reform	Total Quality Management Malcolm Baldridge Tool	Post Reform
Waste Inequal Access to Care Escalating Costs Harm Unnecessary errors	Leadership Results Strategy Operation Focus Workforce Focus Strategy Development Results	Higher quality Increased patient satisfaction Reduced Waste Sustained System Reduced unnecessary costs More efficient health-care system

Figure 2 - Conceptual framework for value-based health-care reform

This research study rested on a foundation of quality improvement, organizational strategies implemented to optimize quality in care and costs, as well as improve organizational performance. The MBCPE criteria served as a tool to explore the business strategies successful in promoting the goals of value-based health care. The MBCPE framework is comprised of seven constructs with impact on quality, cost, and performance.

Literature reviewed showed the MBCPE influenced business strategies and impact organizational performance (Flynn & Saladin, 2001; NIST, 2008). Across the decades, organizational leaders used the criteria to apply for the MBCPE award, or as a self-assessment to improve operations with satisfactory results. These tools can guide organizational leaders as they transition to value-based health care to promote the principles of Total Quality Management (TQM) and consequently sustained organizational excellence.

Organization of the Remainder of the Study

This research was comprised of five chapters. Chapter 1 presented the research problem, the study's purpose, and its significance. A discussion of the assumptions and limitations followed.

Chapter 2 presented a literature review of the need for reform, a brief history of quality in health care, and current efforts to improve. The chapter presented critical information regarding success in value-based health care; comments on missing gaps in academic literature; the applicability of using the MBCPE as a tool for succeeding in value-based health care, and summarized key points and concepts.

Contained in Chapter 3 was a description of the exploratory qualitative inquiry methodology used in this research study. A detailed description of the research design, population, sample framework, sample, sample size, and research instrument was provided. Also included were the researcher background, data collection methods, field testing, and data analysis. A discussion of the validity, credibility, and ethical considerations of the study concluded the chapter.

Presented in Chapter 4 was an outline of the research study, a description of the participant sample, and included secondary data. The next section followed with data analysis of primary and secondary data, categorical aggregation of the data, and data results. Chapter 5 provided a discussion of the study's findings, the implications, conclusions based on results including recommendations for future research in the study of value-based health care.

Chapter 2

Literature Review

At the time of the literature review, there was an absence of research pertaining to the business strategies that facilitated success in value-based health care. A review of the literature identified using the Baldrige Criteria for Performance Excellence (MBCPE) as a quality improvement tool that supported this researcher's study.

Chapter two included an overview of the need to reform health care practices. The literature review presented a historic review of quality improvement concepts, efforts of reform in health care in 2013, and value-based health care. An overview of the issue of measurement of quality outcome was an indicator to quality performance in value-based health care, and its effect on success in value-based program. Following the overview, there was a discussion of the benefit of total quality management as an appropriate theoretical framework to enhance the success of the 2013 value-based health care initiative. Next was a discussion of the suitability of the use of the MBCPE as an operational tool to facilitate application of total quality management principles as a conceptual framework. The intent was not only to use the MBCPE to enhance the business goals of value-based health care, but also as a means for continued organizational excellence and sustainability. The chapter concluded with a summary of key points in the literature review.

The Need for Reform

The United States health-care system contains capabilities via advances in technology, medicine, and evidence-based practices; however, research characterized the system as inefficient, fragmented, and ineffective (Kohn et al., 2001). Issues identified were unequal use of resources, lack of access to care, unnecessary death(s) from errors or complications, and a decreased focus on the patient. The literature highlighted the work of professionals using technological advances to improve the care of services provided and ultimately sustained quality of life for patients. Research showed the system was not producing the outcomes expected from such a technologically advanced system and there was doubt about the overall improvement of quality within the health-care system.

Not only was there evidence of continued waste, disparities in access to care, and unnecessary errors – some resulting in fatalities, but also health-care costs continued to soar and contribute to excessive expenditures for the Medicare program.

National medical and health-care costs are projected to increase to 21% by 2023. Resources dedicated to health care do not commensurate with the dollars spent for the quality of the outcomes. The significance with the pace set in the first decade of the 21st century indicated the United States would not be able to sustain the (current) health system (Baicker & Chandra, 2009; Champy & Greenspun, 2010; Toussaint, 2009). Although advanced treatments increased survival rates and extended patients' lives, the research confirmed the need for reform to transform the delivery and quality of care; the expectation was an increase in quality services provided would reduce unnecessary costs and curb excessive expenditures. By 2013, progress remained slow in the achievement of an efficient and effective system that did not harm, but also improved the quality-of-life for patients.

One of the major problems in health care was the mismanagement of resources – including overuse and underuse. Research showed misuse of resources was the main contributor of waste, inefficiency, ineffectiveness, and did not result in a greater quality of life (Chassin & Galvin, 1998; Kohn et al., 2001; Orszag, 2008). Chassin and Galvin (1998) defined underuse as "the failure to provide a health-care service when it would have produced a favorable outcome for a patient" (p. 1002). Misuse of resources severely affected quality outcomes and costs in the health-care system.

Underuse could often result in health-care disparities for those without insurance or in low, socio-economic areas whom had unequal access to medical and health-care services. Examples of underuse were inadequate treatment, failure to appropriately treat diseases, and rationing of services for patients in need and whom may have benefited from such health-care services (Braveman, Cubbin, Egerter, Williams, & Pamuk, 2010; Reinier et al., 2011). Underuse could severely degrade the quality of life of a patient, especially those in underprivileged classes, and could lead to severe consequences such as death.

Issues of unequal access to care and underuse of resources were another growing major concern within the health-care industry per the literature review. Unequal access greatly affected the value of service provided to the patient, as well as quality of outcomes. Quinn et al. (2011) examined the access to care for those with influenza exposure and found evidence that disparities existed because of poverty-related issues in ethnic groups of Hispanics and African Americans; notably access to treatment was significantly lower in Hispanics and African Americans than in it was in Caucasians. As a result, the perception was there was an increased risk for exposure to influenza – despite nationwide availability of treatment options – and the underuse of health care medical resources because of socio-economic status. Quinn et al. (2011) confirmed results of an earlier study by Linn, Guralnik, and Patel (2010) who initially found unequal access attributable to distribution of influenza treatment because of socio-economic status. McWilliams, Meara, Zaslavsky, and Ayanian (2009) researched cardiovascular disease and diabetes between 1999 and 2006 based on a research study of socio-demographic status. McWilliams et al. found evidence that, although disease control improved over the time-period, inequities in disease control related to race, ethnic, and socio-economic status persisted. These findings were of concern, especially in a health care and medical system that promised to 'do no harm,' and the health care available had the capability of improving and extending patients' lives.

In addition to evidence of underuse, research illustrated a chronic misuse of health care resources that influenced future outcomes for patients. Chassin and Galvin (1998) defined misuse as, "when an appropriate service has been selected, but a preventable complication occurs, and the patient does not receive the full potential of the benefit of the service" (p. 1002). Although a majority of the related-literature research focused on socio-economic status as a reason for underuse, other issues that resulted from inappropriate use of resources included a lack of knowledge of the appropriate services to bring about satisfactory health-care outcomes. Accelerating factors of misuse of health resources often led to a preventable condition or complications such as pneumonia or even death.

Another issue of misuse is overuse. Overuse occurred when a patient receives a battery of services (normally) unwarranted for treatment of the symptoms observed. In the research study to investigate the state of overuse in health-care industry, Korenstein, Falk, Howell, Bishop, and Keyhani (2012) found inappropriate use of antibiotics for treatment of upper-respiratory infections and cardiovascular services, despite universally-accepted guidelines for treatment and intervention. Korenstein et al. also noted an under-emphasis in research of overuse of resources compared to the research available on misuse and underuse of health care resources. Korenstein et al. offered a possible explanation for the lack of evidence of overuse ... as the practice of defensive medicine, a culture that prevails in the health-care system.

A culture of defensive medicine practice is one where practitioners believe more health-care services are better. Promotion of additional services is not in the interest to serve the patient, but to protect providers from litigation. In a practice of defensive medicine, professionals perform or use extra services to maintain relations with the patient, referring providers, or try to mitigate malpractice suits (Hermer & Brody, 2010). To save themselves from litigation, practitioners ignore the possibilities of alternatives that could potentially produce the same or better outcomes. In a study by Nahed, Babu, Smith, and Heary (2012) of more than 1,000 neurosurgeons, 72% of respondents perceived there was a malpractice risk, which led physicians to be more defensive in their medical practice. Providers ordered multiple studies, such as diagnostic testing, to negate a presumed and assumed legal risk. Providers engaged in this behavior, regardless of the reality of the potential gain, risk, loss of reimbursement amounts, or socio-economic status of patient.

Unnecessary services increased costs, and could contribute to decreased attention to a treatment plan relevant to the patient's needs. This practice reduced care provided more than the 'true' value of care, where it was not so much the result of the fear of litigation or use of technology ... it was that the provider did what they felt was appropriate and efficient. Nahed et al. (2012) reported that even though some patients may benefit from cranial procedures, some neurosurgeons have eliminated high-risk procedures, (including cranial procedures), to protect themselves from malpractice suits, as well as avoid medical blame for critical side effects such as paralysis. Nahed et al. reported approximately 45% of respondents simply did not treat high-risk procedures. These actions reduced their litigation potential, but it further reduced access to care of possible life-saving, health care interventions.

A contrasting attitude was that more advanced and invasive health care treatments were better, regardless of the potential for debilitating, physical side effects. Although providers may not agree with this logic, they could be at risk for ridicule from their peers or dissatisfaction from their patients (Evans, Thornton, Chalmers, & Glasziou, 2011). Providers did not practice or consider appropriate use of resources for the most efficient or effective path to an increased quality of life for the patient. The collective effect of a defensive culture was exacerbated via misuse and/or overuse created a system plagued with deficiencies, inefficiencies, and reduced health-care service capabilities. If this behavior continues, it could lead to negative, national financial consequences and reduced quality of life for some patients.

A component of the high quality of health care was using the appropriate resources to provide the necessary health-care treatment(s). Providing the most appropriate health-care services could promote holistic wellness and give patients a better quality of life. AHRQ provided a systematic definition stating, "quality health care means striking the right balance of [health care] service by avoiding underuse, overuse, and eliminating misuse" (Clancy, 2005, p. 3). High quality of health care means processes within the system would be error free, non-wasteful, and achieve the desired results for the patient, as well as a balance of financial stability and quality services for the organization. The AHRQ summed up components of quality by stating quality is "doing the right thing, at the right time, in the right way, for the right person, to achieve the best possible results" (Hibbard & Sofaer, 2010, Model Report, para. 1). The fundamentals of quality were necessary to prevent overburdening the national budget and a breakdown of the system's capabilities to increase patients' health. The idea of fundamentals of quality initiated efforts were those that drew attention to the patient, the process, the outcomes, and the payment. Determination of the best business strategies to health-care services improvement was contingent upon the various organizational perspectives of quality.

History of Quality Improvement Strategies

Quality improvement efforts were contingent on the multiple perspectives of quality and therefore led to strategies for improvement. Quality improvement strategies evolved as elements of what constituted quality, such as the patient, the process, or outcomes, and kept shifting. To enable sustained improvement within the health-care industry, it was important to evaluate past concepts of quality improvement and determine practices or strategies to enhance current health care goals and to realize desired levels of quality and efficiency.

Over 150 years ago, the inherent value of professional skill and a focal concern of 'do no harm' formed the basis of the quality of healthcare. Quality improvement pioneers such as Florence Nightingale promoted caring attitudes and behavior as the fundamentals of quality health care. The need to improve and seek better quality practices stemmed from the concerns of professionals who wanted to increase positive medical and health-care outcomes for patients. There was limited literature and historical findings about patients demanding high expectations of quality. The lack of demand may have been from uninformed patients whom did not believe they had a choice to demand quality in health care (Komashie, Mousavi, & Gore, 2007). Although patients did not know they had a choice to demand quality, the expectation was the health-care providers were giving the patients the best possible care, via the providers' medical ethics, the health-care providers did so.

Over the last two decades (previous to the date gathered within this research study), attitudes shifted from medical and health-care providers' desire to improve standards of quality because of ethical concerns to do better for patients, to motives based on monetary value and 'beating' the competition. The reason for this shift in the medical industry was researchers found that improvements in organizational activities led to an increase in profits and a competitive position for organizations. In 2013, improvement efforts no longer solely highlighted the ethical obligation to help the patient, but included an emphasis for organizational activities such as clinical and business within organizations that increased both profits and patient satisfaction.

Quality pioneers such as Shewhart, Donabedian, Deming, Juran, and Crosby offered perceptions of systematic quality improvement methods and developed frameworks regarding quality improvement strategies based on these perceptions (Suarez, 1992). Quality improvement pioneers' goals were to retain customers through satisfaction of a high-quality product (or service). The business focus was on the production of a high-quality product and improvement of the process within the organization. Unlike Florence Nightingale's belief of caring behaviors as the ethical foundation to quality in health care, who's views were more systematic, pioneer health-care providers' views were more systematic, and research provided more influence on quality, in addition to 'caring behaviors.'

Quality improvement concepts were primarily developed for manufacturing industries, but eventually gained recognition in the health-care industry resulting in the potential to decrease costs and increase client (patient) loyalty.

Previous quality improvement strategies focused on organizational activities such as process improvement, satisfaction, and the final product or service; the strategies were developed to help improve the competitive position and, therefore, profits. Quality improvement in health care incorporated concepts of leadership, knowledge management, measurement, and commitment to quality improvement. Despite the lack of a confirmed universal definition of quality, varied quality definitions and quality improvement frameworks cumulatively shared underlying principles of customer satisfaction, the need for a solid product, and an evaluation of processes to ensure delivery a product that was essentially defect-free. Shewhart (1931), a seminal thinker of quality improvement, presented the impact of processes on consumer's needs and on the quality of products as a systematic means of quality improvement. Shewhart defined quality in terms of how the product was constituted, that is, from its objective inherent characteristics, as well as the customer's subjective view of the product's characteristics. Shewhart believed it necessary to adapt organizational processes to ensure the product characteristics create satisfactory outcomes.

Shewhart (1931) believed appropriate steps to workflow improvement created a well-manufactured product, rather than to wait to inspect the product at the end of the manufacturing process. His greatest contribution was the Plan-Do-Check-Act cycle also known as the Shewhart cycle used to help an organization's leadership understand the productivity of their organizational processes and develop steps for improvement. Shewhart deemed it necessary to have constant evaluation of practices to ensure managers make appropriate and timely decisions. Shewhart also emphasized the need for management to commit to constant evaluation and make timely and appropriate business decisions; the focus of his model was on the processes that impacted the product outcomes. Shewhart did not take into consideration other influential factors other than process, for example, the impact of each employee's responsibility for producing products and services.

Leaders could design processes to be efficient; however, to achieve desired outcomes, the reviewed literature revealed the whole organizations should be committed and accept responsibility for outcomes. Blumenthal and Kilo (1998) stressed the importance of organizing and preparing projects, so staff are not overwhelmed, and to not view efforts of improvement as just another fad. It was necessary to consider other business influences in improving quality outcomes.

While Shewhart (1931) highlighted the need to ensure efficient processes to ensure production of satisfactory outcomes, Donabedian (2005) proposed evaluation of quality from a model incorporating more than the process. Donabedian used three categories: structure, process, and outcome to assess quality. Donabedian's model of structure, process, and outcome(s) grouped more organizational activities into three separate categories for implementation of strategies for improvement. Structure refers to 1) availability and accessibility of resources (e.g., staff, equipment, and other organizational characteristics); 2) process as the delivery of health care described by what the technical and interpersonal processes do (or fail to do), and 3) the final products of health care, such as quality of life and health status as outcomes. (Donabedian, 2005). Donabedian's (2005) believed the health-care structure was the driving force for successful health-care institutions' organizational processes and outcomes, because care is structurally organized. Variability in the structure of organizations could affect the quality of care delivered. This model's goals were for accountability and proper management of care that addressed key elements affecting health care outcomes. Donabedian's concept resulted in the implementation of accreditation and regulation initiatives. The model was popular and served as a basis for quality improvement in health-care organizations, especially as it included multiple facets of the organization (e.g., human resources, training, patient care and treatment, patient satisfaction, and the facility itself. Donabedian's model may continue to be beneficial in today's environment, especially used in collaboration with other models.

    While Donabedian's model considered additional elements of organizational influences on producing quality outcomes, critics argued the model was too linear (sequential) and did not account for evaluation of the influence of each of the categories to each other. Others offered the model did not consider other factors that affect clinical processes and therefore the outcomes. These factors included, patient characteristics or the influence of the internal environment (the context) or the external environment (political or market influence). Another criticism was the structure; Donabedian (2005) described the model as an indirect measure of quality. A reason for this critic's opinion was structural characteristics such as staff, culture, and technology used may have influenced quality of services. According to Cromwell et al. (2011) and Alexander, Hearld, Jiang, and Fraser (2007), structure is an indirect measure of quality, whereas clinical process and outcomes provided a closer representation of true quality. The main strength of Donabedian's model was adaptability to integrate other quality improvement theories for a more holistic strategy for organizations. A framework that could enhance its adaptability and strength is Deming's Total Quality Management (TQM) model.

Deming, a student of Shewhart, added to quality improvement concepts, theorizing that issues of quality were systematic (Spencer, 1994). Deming recognized the need for a strategy that integrated independent elements, e.g., management, market, market research, commitment, documentation, training, and customer, with organizational processes to produce desired outcomes (Asubonteng, McCleary, & Munchus, 1996). These factors directly influenced subsequent processes that achieved desired results.

Deming's idea incorporated more elements of organizational activities that can be considered an expansion or deviation of Donabedian's structure category. Deming focused on a broader scope of 'structure' he believed impacted processes to produce desirable outcomes. Deming postulated that quality was a never-ending cycle and a journey that an organization undertakes as opposed to a static process.

"The focus is on the preservation and health of the organization, but there also are explicitly stated values about the organization's context (the community and customers) and about the well-being of individual organization members" (Hackman & Wageman, 1995, p. 310). Deming's model provided a multi-faceted approach that addressed more than one area within an organization. Evaluation of the health-care system would have maintained excellence through a multi-faceted assurance system.

Deming believed quality perceptions change according to the needs of the customer. To Deming, a key characteristic in quality improvement is the ability to know when to act and when to leave a process alone based on outcomes desired – quality management. Deming emphasized the importance of integrating quality improvement factors into facilitated organizations to focus on business practice and management efforts to improve processes, to reduce costs, as well as cost variabilities, to produce satisfactory outcomes, e.g., unnecessary costs, improved care delivery, patient satisfaction, reduced delays in diagnosis, and appropriate treatment.

In contrast to Deming's broader view, but more relevant approach, to quality improvement, Juran's (1993) definition and framework of quality stressed the importance of satisfying the customer as a quality outcome. Juran defined quality in terms of customer satisfaction. Juran believed products should possess limited deficiencies. Organizations needed proper strategy formulation to ensure the processes delivered products that satisfied the customer (Asubonteng et al., 1996; Suarez, 1992). Focusing on the processes within the organization is an important business concept within the health-care organization. Juran directed leaders to identify and strategize the health-care delivery processes needed to ensure customer satisfaction. There was a flaw in Juran's quality model. Leaders must possess knowledge and skill sets to identify the process improvement strategies that would have provided positive benefits to the organization or institution; otherwise these leaders were left to guess at what will work, which can consume unnecessary resources.

Although Juran (1993) emphasized defect-free products, Crosby (1992) highlighted the importance of *limited deficiencies* in the processes that deliver the product or service. Crosby, another quality pioneer known for his 'zero defects' philosophy, shared similar, but contrasting, views with Juran. Crosby's focus was to prevent process deficiencies (zero defects) and limit variance in quality as opposed to a definition of strategies to improve products in case the outcomes were defective. Although there are benefits associated with such strategies, reduction in waste is only one component of quality improvement. Despite Crosby's specific focus on preventing process deficiencies, and thus waste reduction, he noted the importance of organization culture was key to implementing quality improvement and other ideas similar to Deming. Crosby and Juran, like Shewhart, failed to discuss the effect of additional factors on their model(s), for example, untrained employees. Untrained employees would interfere with organizations attaining full benefits from their models that contributed toward sustained quality and excellence. To realize substantial improvements in health care, a model that addresses various facets of organization functions was both crucial and beneficial to producing satisfactory outcomes.

Shewhart, Donabedian, Deming, Juran, and Crobsy provided concepts that, integrated as a collaborative model, could improve efficiency in the United States' business – or health-care – industry. Despite varied perspectives, Shewhart, Deming, and Juran argued costs would decrease as quality increased, because products would be delivered right the first time; the quality process eliminated the need for re-work. Demand for products would increase and require lower production costs, resulting in higher performance and financial profits. Shewhart, Deming, and Juran's efforts focused on streamlining production, reducing human error, emphasizing the importance of commitment to quality improvement, and using data to drive decision-making (Alexander & Hearld, 2009; Luce, Bindman, & Lee, 1994). Quality process elements (streamlining, reduction of errors, commitment to quality), according to the literature on business excellence, were important for maintenance of a highly efficient organization. Despite evidence, efforts to improve via quality assurance processes are yet to sustain desired levels of health-care services and process improvement for quality of life for patients. Progress was slow and with the impact of the recession on national finances; the government revisited the need for reform.

Previous Efforts

In the past, organizations used various quality improvement strategies such as Lean Six Sigma, benchmarking, restructuring, and supply-chain management to address deficiencies within health-care systems or to improve efficiency and better clinical quality and financial outcomes. Although these strategies provided improved process benefits, none sustained improvement within the health-care industry. Early efforts to improve quality outcomes were only in the interest of the organization to maintain a competitive edge or adhere to accreditation standards. Those health-care organizations who had the financial resources to dedicate to enhancing their competitive edge and profits voluntarily sought improvement measures to become better at delivering quality care ... and ultimately ... more financially stable than the competition. Health-care organizations using quality improvement methods that minimized costs of health-care interventions realized greater profits, rather than solely maximizing the value of care during the patient care cycle.

Past efforts by health-care organizations also focused on shifting costs, capturing the competition's revenue, and adding more health-care services as methods to increase revenue and to remain financially sustainable (Porter, 2009). Porter warned that setting goals without emphasizing value could lead to dangerous, false, and self-defeating outcomes.

Porter blamed failure of health-care reform efforts, as previous health-care improvement goals did not emphasize value as the underlying driver for health improvement. These improvement efforts did not emphasize the value of care to the patient as the focus was on profits – not on delivering the best care per dollar spent.

Lack of Encouragement

In the past, little legal impetus occurred to encourage quality improvement efforts mainly in terms of reducing unnecessary costs primarily, because of opposition from key persons who were at risk for losing income. No real incentive existed for meaningful change to evaluate critically and change habits, especially for those lagging in health-care quality improvement; nor was there an industry commitment to translate interest in quality improvement strategies effectively in the health-care organization.

Marmor, Oberlander, and White (2009) blamed the political structure of the health-care system as a deterrent in containing expenditures, as implied in a reduction in income for key-investment stockholders, such as insurance companies. Marmor et al. speculated this was the reason for the neglect and opposition of the health-care reforms, especially curtailing costs for health-care institutions, initially proposed by Presidents Nixon and Clinton. Because of this reform opposition in 2013, the government had yet to control rising health-care costs. Inability to curtail costs was possibly because of the recession, when the impact of cost control deficiencies of the system became more urgent to address by the government.

The Institute of Medicine (IOM) blamed the design, processes, and capabilities of the health-care system and suggested a redesign that focused on leadership engagement, use of quality measurement tools, and quality improvement protocols to reduce defects, increase of transparency, and increase the standardization of health-care processes and patient quality outcomes (Kohn et al., 2001). A redesign of the health-care system would aid in the reduction of the unproductive work habits and will alleviate the cost burden by reducing unnecessary medical procedures, eliminating the need for additional services resulting from errors, and potential increasing the quality of life for the patient.

Despite theories of quality improvement strategies and evidence to support such strategies, holistic quality improvement remains evasive. A possible reason for this failure was limited legal incentive to curb the unproductive habits. Blumental and Kilo (1998) reported that leaders who experimented with quality improvement (QI) strategies lost their enthusiasm after these strategies did not meet expectations or provided unsatisfactory results. There were no incentives to improve … the organization received payment regardless of the quality of their healthcare services and patient outcomes. Blame for failed health-care QI reform efforts cannot rest on organizations' leadership. The nation's political environment heavily influenced the state of the health-care industry. Government and private payers reimbursed organizations for services, regardless of their unproductive habits, poor quality outcomes, and/or disparities in health care and related access to medical facilities.

Payment Reform

Poor quality not only affects patients, but also payers of health care. The evidence from previous landmark studies that highlighted problems of medical errors, safety, excessive costs, and quality of care helped initiate new governmental policies regarding improving quality and developing financial incentives for improvement through pay-for-performance (Chassin et al., 2010; Kohn et al., 2001; Wachter, 2004). Although the current definition of quality focuses on efficiency and effectiveness (and therefore on payment reform), healthcare reform policies should bring about radical improvement/ improved outcomes by reducing the misuse of resources and increasing the value of delivered health care. The idea behind reform is to change attitudes and be of service to others, that is, focus on the value of care provided. Previous attitudes of earning revenue through volume only increased the nation's issues of poor quality, disparities in health care access, and excessive costs. To change these non-caring attitudes, payers of health-care services also proposed models of reform to focus on increasing the value of services provided through more patient-centric care and accountability in practice. Medicare took on pecuniary measures of motivation.

The notion behind this pecuniary measure, or value-based care, is that if payments are contingent on specific clinical indicators or outcomes, then providers will be forced and/or encouraged to perform at their best to deliver efficient and effective care (Greene, 2009; McIntyre, Rogers, & Heier, 2001; Rosenthal & Frank, 2006). Organizations will have to evaluate health-care delivery systems to make appropriate choices to facilitate quality in outcomes per dollars spent. In 2013, reimbursements were contingent – not on the service(s) medical providers provided – but on how well organizations provided services and the sustained outcome that resulted in improved quality of life for the patient.

Current Efforts

As previous quality improvement strategies did not sustain improvement, possibly because of the traditional fee-based service payment methods, issues of poor quality persist. Under the Patient Protection and Affordable Care Act (2010), Medicare launched a revised pay-for-performance (PFP) program, more commonly referred to as value-based care. The premise of the PFP program was that withholding payments unless clinical outcomes are met would reduce unnecessary health care expenditures and encourage health-care provider organizations to operate efficiently and effectively as high-performance systems. It is the government's intent to hold health-care provider organizations financially accountable for quality patient care and treatment outcomes. Medicare's approach was instrumental in realizing change ... not only in containing costs ...but in improving quality through emphasizing the value of the care provided.

Medicare withholds (punitive) payments to hospitals by an estimated $964 million, or one percent of reimbursements amount (CMS, 2012). The amount of money withheld is based on the quality of its care determined through established criteria; organizations must deliver a high quality of care and sustain quality practices to ensure maximum reimbursement. Based on previous research, Medicare chose 12 clinical measures and eight patient experience measures as indicators for quality patient outcomes. The 12 clinical measures are in the areas of heart attack, heart failure, hospital acquired infection, pneumonia, surgical care improvement measures; claims-based measures (mortality and readmissions); healthcare-associated infections measures; surgical complications measure; patient experience of care survey-based measure; immunization measures; and structural measures to assess hospitals' capacity to improve quality of care.

Eight patient experiences of care measures exist in the areas of nurse, doctor, and medication communication: hospital staff responsiveness, pain management, hospital cleanliness, discharge information, and overall hospital rating, which are grouped under the Hospital Consumer Assessment of Healthcare Providers and Systems Survey ([HCAHPS] CMS, 2013). The drive to increase patient satisfaction had become an industry-wide effort. HCAHPS reporting is public information and a tool to help patients compare hospital experiences of past and current patients' ratings measuring one facility against other hospitals in the geographic. Other goals, as published by the U.S. Department of Health and Human Services (2011) outlined by The National Quality Strategy to improve the health-care system, include the following:

> *Better Care: improve the overall quality, by making health care more patient-centered, accessible, and safe.*
>
> *Healthy People/Healthy Communities: improve the health of the U.S. population by supporting proven interventions to address behavioral, social, and environmental determinants of health in addition to delivering higher-quality care.*

Affordable Care: reduce the cost of quality health care for individuals, families, employers, and government (p. 1).

The disadvantage of previous efforts by health-care organizations was shifting away from servicing patients' needs and producing better outcomes that improved the patient's quality of life, and therefore increasing overall patient satisfaction. Tralib and Rahman (2010) stated that customer satisfaction was the essence of long-term organizational success, and it was important to understand customers' needs through patient feedback. In 2013, efforts attempted to re-shift the focus on the customer for the reason Tralib and Rahman suggested, as well as ethical obligation to do what is right for the patient. The aims of the pay-for-performance program was to increase quality through clinical practices that prevented patients from becoming ill or suffer complications during treatment while using the most effective and efficient cycle of health care.

Value-based Health Care

As of October 2012, value-based, health care was the new method of quality and payment reform by Medicare to promote higher quality in health-care services, which subsequently should have lowered costs. Economic theory hypothesized linking payments to performance would entice health-care provider organizations to change their patterns of behavior (Prendergast, 1999). The underlying principle is transforming the payment system from one that paid based on volume of services to one that pays based on the value of care delivered for the money spent would have enhanced and reached the goals of cost efficiency and care effectiveness. Value-based care differs from previous improvement attempts, because the underlying principles were placed on efficiency, cost containment, and increased quality; the underlying causes of system deficiencies related to misuse of organizational resources and poor outcomes for both patient and organization were addressed. The value-based care initiative had the potential to lower excessive expenditures, consume fewer resources, and increase the quality of care delivered, which ultimately led to a better quality of life and health-care outcomes via better quality of health care for patients.

Medicare officials chose to incentivize payments based on common clinical conditions associated with the highest revenue costs. Officials chose these areas because of potential complications that could result from treatment or the potential to acquire an infection during treatment stay and, thus, more likely to impact patient outcomes. In 2013, the effort of reform is dedicated to the patient population who received the most expensive care. The Medicare program expended resources for the people the entity served. Medicare reported about 15% of Medicare patients experienced an adverse event during hospitalization, and about 33% of patients needed re-admission within one month of discharge (VanLare, Moody-Williams, & Conway, 2012).

Adverse events and associated hospital readmissions constituted avoidable health-care costs associated with the quality of health care. Although Schoen (2013) advised it was important to focus on the system and not just the federal reform aspect, it was better to implement reform in the health-care organizations responsible for 40% of the population who receive the highest dollar amount of care. Schoen described payment reform as a method to "accelerate the pace of delivery system innovation, care integration, and coordination, while increasing accountability for improving outcomes and reducing cost growth per beneficiary over time" (p. 22). The outcomes of value-based health care had the potential to accomplish changes for an enhanced health-care system. Given the history of failed attempts at establishing sustained health-care reform, value-based care offered a solution for addressing issues that continued to plague the health-care industry.

The goals of value-based health care, according to Medicare, enhanced the quality of care through an emphasis on the value of care provided specifically in several clinical areas identified by Medicare (CMS, 2013). According to Medicare, increased quality in these areas not only contributed to better quality outcomes for patient, but also can significantly reduce expenditures for the organization. This reduction was because of fewer complications or reduced adverse events (e.g., acquiring conditions not present when originally admitted). Organizations must significantly improve in these areas, as Stone et al. (2010) reported. Preventable adverse events, more commonly referred to as hospital associated infections, are the sixth leading cause of death in the United States and annually resulted in almost $50B in unnecessary expenses.

Hospital readmissions, another clinical measure exert costs of over $12B annually (Jencks, Williams, & Coleman, 2009). Organizations received points and, ultimately, reimbursement money based on improvements in these newly imposed health-care measures. The industry should see a considerable improvement in quality of patient care outcomes and a reduction in unnecessary expenditures as organizations gain an increased desire to quality ensure health-care service performance, equal to or exceeding Medicare requirements, to remain financial viable. Organizations will not receive reimbursement for these conditions if the outcomes are not in alignment with those proposed by the Centers for Medicare and Medicaid Services (CMS) (Hines & Yu, 2009). To ensure health-care organizations receive the maximum reimbursement, organizations need to redefine clinical approaches to patient are to ensure health-care organizations deliver value at the lowest cost.

Between health systems, a fierce competition exists around these metrics, and with decreasing reimbursement from the payer, it places a strong incentive on continuously improving the level and quality of care delivered. In 2013, quality of care included the patients' perceptions of their care plan as well. Medicare makes payments based on the health-care organization's performance or improved performance in each clinical measure during a baseline period (CMS, 2011). These measures target roughly 3,500 hospitals in the United States. Over the next few years (after the publication of this research study; 2013-2018)< the pay-for-performance program will extend slowly to other types of organizations such as free-standing / independent clinics. Medicare anticipated that increased attention to performance in clinical areas will provide a potential solution quality deficiencies within the health-care system, especially costs and quality of patient care delivered. Organizations should redefine approaches to clinical quality improvement to realize success in pay-for-performance program.

Given the financial pressures and the need to contain costs, value-based health care can be considered a modern necessity that provides the best solution to ensure improvement in the quality of care delivered as well as a reduction in health care expenditures. Organizational health-care leaders can benefit from implementing strategies to realize success in the program. Leaders need to find ways to manage their clinical and financial resources to reduce costs and increase the value of services provided. Roland (2012) stated, "Pay-for-performance is not a new drug that will cure the quality problems in contemporary health-care systems; however, it has a place, yet to be fully defined, in our armamentarium" (p. 913 Medicare's program cannot be successful if the program only addresses clinical aspects and not the entire system. Lack of information about the non-clinical aspects can hinder an organization's efforts of improvement.

Efficacy of Value-based Care

To redefine business approaches, attitudes toward elements of health care and quality of patient care sustainability need to change. Attitude based on recognizing the value in services provided was not intrinsic to the system, because previous initiatives of improvements were focused on increasing profits through volume. In 2013, the health-care industry attitude was to stress value versus volume; and supposedly would help alleviate the financial burden the health-care industry placed on the national budget. Mehrotra, Damberg, Melony, Sorbero, and Teleki (2009) were doubtful of the true impact of the value-based care to improving system deficiencies. Mehrotra et al. stated, although claims of cost savings and effectiveness of care were made, the results of the three-year experimentation by Medicare were not published. These authors believed there was unnecessary enthusiasm for value-based care. Mehrotra et al. stated the lack of evidence or the small improvement in quality previous studies had found; value-based care can have unintended consequences, such as medical professionals caring for healthier and more compliant patients to ensure performance outcomes are met and ultimately not having reimbursements withheld.

In previous studies, the empirical foundation of payers providing reimbursement based on the value of care as measured by performance outcomes was mixed. In Mehrotra et al.'s (2009) study, over 50% reported a return on investment on money spent when complying with the Medicare program. Mehrotra et al. indicated that despite a positive response to reimbursements based on performance, continued work existed in refining the program to bring about higher gains. Other studies by Werner and McNutt (2009) and Borden (2012) provided guidance for improvement in achieving desired levels of outcomes and not in terms of the process of strategies that could achieve maximum reimbursement. Leaders may not have been aware of types of business strategies in employee development, strategy development, and decision-making that worked best to achieve desired outcomes, because additional influences may have helped determine root causes of poor quality.

Quality improvement in health care was an evolving and dynamic process, but it is important to identify a framework to guide actions toward improvement. Werner, Kolstad, Stuart, and Polsky (2011) noted little is known on how to use a value-based program effectively. Werner et al. concluded that for Medicare's program to work, organizations must tailor the program concepts to suit the health-care organizations situation. Werner et al. stated more research must address design and implementation of the program to enhance its effectiveness. Marmor and Oberlander (2011) argued the cost initiatives associated with value-based health care is "akin to throwing darts" (p. 481). Oberlander and Marmor argued the need for payment reform, considering other countries (e.g., Canada) uses a fee-for-service system, and has better cost control than the United States. Oberlander and Marmor argued the United States should be emulating Canadian policies; not trying to reinvent and reorganize solution to the problems.

Despite this speculation, Medicare officials firmly believed the pay-for-performance program was likely to transform attitudes toward the delivery of quality heath care. In 2013, fee-for-performance remains a plausible solution, especially in comparison to the resulting issues of overuse and misuse of using the traditional fee-for-service payment program.

Medicare viewed the pay-for-performance initiative with optimism, particularly concerning potential costs savings and improvement in the quality of life for patients. Several problems may affect the long-term success of the pay-for-performance initiative. These problems include health-care organizations engaging in primary practices to receive and ensure reimbursements rather than engaging in total organization transformation. While value-based initiatives may be the only solution, more research is needed for comprehensive results … that is, aside from the clinical improvements. There were no evidence-based guidelines or theories found in this researcher's literature review available to assist organizational leaders fully understand how to transition from a fee-for-service industry and thrive in a value-based one.

Problems with Current Efforts

The lack of a comprehensive approach to value-based care would be a reason for the mixed results of studies evaluating the impact of payment based on performance. Those characteristics of value-based care only addressed performance in the clinical areas measured. The final improved clinical outcomes could not be the main indicator of quality improvement. It would be impossible for health-care organizations to be successful in the pay-for-performance program with just a guideline of clinically-desired outcomes. A focus on specific quality measures may not provide the broader quality result the health-care system needs (Werner, Bradlow, & Asch, 2008). Heffner, Mularski, and Calverley (2010) shared similar views that some aspects of clinical care may be under-represented by quality measures and sufficient resources may not be devoted to the areas of clinical care not specified by Medicare's program care. Heffner et al. stated the lack of a system-wide program might contribute to worsening of the quality assurance of patient health care. Health care is a complex entity with many influencing factors, so it seemed impossible to achieve satisfactory outcomes in specific clinical areas to increase overall quality and performance through the health-care organization, let alone the entire health-care industry.

In 2013, the challenges with achieving performance outcomes in value-based care were unknown regarding which approach is appropriate or will be best suited for the organization. As a result, organizations had to work backward based on the outcomes of clinical goals to determine strategies to produce positive outcomes, rather than working from a better aligned strategic business plan to bring about such outcomes at the onset of planning and developing. Some organizations may not have the knowledge, the time, or the resources to dedicate to developing a more aligned strategy. Leaders are left to guess methods that work or on which areas to focus, and hope the quality improvement methods they chose would increase accountability, improve the care delivered, reduce unnecessary costs, and deliver the quality of care expected to earn the organization's Medicare invoice reimbursements. Leaders may devise inappropriate strategies (as they failed to consider the business impact or structure of the organization and its influence) on processes to achieve desired outcomes. Therefore, random devising of strategies may not be the answer to support quality improvement changes. To bring about significant change, organizations should focus first on the structural factors to include organizational environment that affect quality issues and, second, to employ a comprehensive tool to address help resolve or curb issues that contributed to unsatisfactory quality practices and uncontrollable expenditures.

As a mean to achieve holistic improvement in the industry, it is necessary to recognize and analyze the root causes of variability. Managers can undertake appropriate actions to improve clinical and business processes to achieve patient care and financial desired outcomes. Lukas et al. (2007) advised that to effectively to bring about change, the elements of the change initiative needs alignment with both the clinical and the business. The elements of value-based care are focused on the outcomes. Heffner et al. (2010) proposed, that though performance measures are important tools, more research is needed to determine underlying hidden consequences leading to poor outcomes. Lack of knowledge in specific areas to improve may contribute to an increase in health delivery disparities between organizations and an increased risk of financial disaster for the organization resulting from lack of Medicare invoice reimbursement. Organizations may continue to deliver poor health care from factors that negatively influence business outcomes. Organizations should have knowledge of business strategies that work best. Though experiences are essential to the learning process, a haphazard approach can be costly, time consuming, and can place an organization in financial distress.

Regardless of the lack of knowledge of non-clinical performance measures in value-based care, the literature reiterates superior quality results from sustained business and clinical excellence. A solution to the holistic problem is to structure the value-based initiative to include both clinical and non-clinical business measures. The focus should be the business strategic path for improvement processes to achieving outcomes, including business processes. Eijkenaar (2012) offered that limiting incentives to specific aspects of care may result in neglect in the other aspects of care. Eijkenaar believed the structure of the pay-for-performance program is critical to a health-care organization's success. Eijkenaar (2012) and Mehrotra et al. (2009) concluded a lack of evidence exists to support successful designs. Mehrotra et al. criticized the use of a limited number of clinical conditions to evaluate the impact of pay-for-performance on improved quality.

This researcher found sparse literature and empirical studies investigating the financial consequences and the impact of business strategies underlying value-based health care practices, the industry can benefit from additional research studies and literature on the positive impact of the elements of TQM on quality and sustained business excellence, to devise and implement strategies accordingly. The amount of literature is vast in 'general' quality improvement. Buttell, Hendler, and Daley (2008) offered that achieving high quality did not have to be challenging. According to Buttell et al., success in achieving high quality was possible if key concepts of quality were identified and understood.

To bring about the changes needed in health care, Kumar et al. (2011) offered that the necessity of improving the system through an integration of resources; for example, increasing efficiency in staff, using resources such as technology, understanding consumer behavior, and evaluating hospital, insurance, and provider costs. Berwick, Nolan, and Whittington (2008) also offered that components of health care goals are dependent on each other. Yaacob (2010) confirmed Jayamaha, Grigg, and Mann's (2008) findings on the critical factors of TQM such as customer focus, leadership, and teamwork impacts the performance of an organization must work synergistically to bring about increased quality in performance and results. Kumar et al. (2011) found these critical factors influence costs, productivity, and the characteristics of products and services. The results also endorsed non-clinical factors as crucial in the quality of clinical outcomes. It is important to acknowledge the impact of the business processes on quality outcomes, so leaders can develop and implement strategies best suited to sustain quality. It is necessary to holistically improve the organization by first linking clinical and non-clinical goals, instead of improving them independently.

For improvement throughout the organization, which eventually will permeate to the industry, organizations must be held accountable for leadership's actions in non-clinical areas. Stone et al. (2009) interviewed 32 participants with industry knowledge, seeking input for strategies that best addressed preventable hospital acquired infections, safety, funding systems, and Medicare policymaking and found additional factors that may impact the effect of pay-for-performance. These variables included leadership behaviors that drove culture change, staff behavior, predisposing patient factors, and regulatory factors that influenced outcomes.

Despite this finding, little attention was paid to the business strategies essential to achieving the quality outcomes in critical clinical areas identified as essential elements of improvement. Literature and empirical studies were sparse in investigating the financial consequences and the impact of business strategies underlying value-based health care practices.

In a literature review of studies performed from 1980-2005, Beauvais and Wells (2006) found most research focused on clinical outcomes and not on financial or other business factors. With operational complexities, already in health-care organizations, leaders may face the problem of not knowing how to achieve these outcomes or may not have the time or resources to experiment with new practices.

Alignment of value-based care initiative to incorporate systemic strategies to achieve the desired outcomes may serve as a more durable and holistic infrastructure to increasing quality.

In 2013, health-care organization's efforts were focused on outcome measures as indicators of quality performance, but outcome measures have implications for achieving limited and specific improvement instead of accomplishing holistic change. Superior quality is not synonymous with specific positive outcomes. Satisfactory outcomes guaranteed neither; data on specific evidence-based interventions were put into action within the organization nor that providers were committed to delivering a high quality of care. The problem with value-based health care is performance rests mainly in the emphasis on health care clinical outcomes. Organizations may be more inclined to focus on specific areas rather than non-clinical elements that contributed to improving overall quality of care. Frustrated leaders sought more methods to improve individual processes rather than address the entire system. Although organizations may have achieved their organization clinical measurement goals, they may not experience sustained clinical quality improvement outcomes.

Proponents of performance measures argued clinical measures outlined by Medicare offer insight to improving most aspects of health care, as well as providing feedback on patients' experiences and their resulting quality of life (Jones, Jones, & Miller, 2004;

Mant, 2001). Performance measures promoted the use of proven treatments that could result in greater benefits to patients. Werner et al. (2008) used the example of administration of fibrinolytic therapy, such as aspirin for a patient with acute myocardial infarction (AMI). These authors theorized success in such measures might also reflect practices that lead to success in areas of unmeasured quality of care. For example, organizations that met the performance measurements and successfully documented administration of aspirin may have had improved levels of unmeasured aspects of care, such as, emergency responsiveness, patient safety, and care coordination. Werner and McNutt (2009) also stated organizations may be at risk for poor healthcare and business outcomes if leaders are inattentive to other outcomes that affected quality. Based on those authors' arguments, clinical-performance measures are not enough to sustain long-term quality improvement.

The argument to support the focus on outcomes as quality performance indicators does not account for patients who may experience satisfactory outcomes despite poor quality, especially if the patients could defeat their disease. Werner et al.'s (2009) study findings suggested improvement in unmeasured aspects of care. For the example provided, there was almost a sequential relationship between emergency responsiveness or care coordination and the delivery of aspirin; hence, results may have shown improvement in those areas.

Werner et al.'s findings did not account for employee expertise on delivering the medication in a timely manner or even the culture of the organization that may or may not display competence in providing health-care services. Werner et al. noted inconsistent findings in similar studies and suggested further research to determine the benefit of using performance measures or assess the quality of outcomes. The researcher found no definite knowledge of or literature reporting whether the effect of pay-for-performance will increase or decrease other clinical outcomes or were measured.

Delivering a high quality of care requires simultaneous efforts of clinical and non-clinical factors. The research shows in addition to clinical outcomes, that error rates, market share, waste, and productivity could also be used as measurements of performance. These factors were components of the TQM, also known as continuous quality improvement (CQI) developed by Deming to improve quality to exceed customer's expectations and maintain organization performance.

Salaheldin (2009), in a study of small and medium businesses in the Qatari industry, confirmed the relationship between TQM and enhanced competitiveness, which supported improved business performance, quality improvement, operation improvement, financial and non-financial business components. Salaheldin's study illustrated non-clinical factors, such as leadership, culture, employee development, and data analysis, did have an influence on the control, design, and use of resources for operational processes, which impacted product or service characteristics. The high-quality characteristics of the products or services contributed to increased revenue and satisfaction from customers. Because of the impact on the outcomes, the study's findings confirmed the significant relationship between the non-clinical factors and organizational performance. Salaheldin's study confirmed earlier studies by Han, Chen, Ebrahimpour, and Sodhi (2001) that found an increase in performance and outcomes resulting from quality management practices. Yeung, Cheng, and Kee-hung (2006) revealed increased performance in their operations, cost-efficiency, customer service, quality, and in profitability compared to those who do not use TQM practices.

A drawback of the value-based care initiative outlined by Medicare was the sole emphasis on achieving target outcomes as an indicator of quality of performance. Such emphasis, according to Werner et al. (2009), captured only one aspect of care: the process of care. This focus implied other aspects of care that could possibly have had an impact on outcomes were overlooked. This omission could lead to issues of misallocation of resources, positive outcomes – despite other issues of poor quality and complete ignorance of additional factors – that impacted the quality of the performance.

The benefit of measures Medicare identified was those measured helped determine if health care provided was good or bad. Without measurement, it was difficult to assess outcomes of the quality of the health care delivered (Leape & Berwick, 2005). Measures could be misunderstood, poorly communicated, and when received by health organizations, may have overlooked underlying issue of poor quality, hence the failure of some quality improvement strategies geared at performance outcomes (Ricondo & Viles, 2005; Werner & McNutt, 2009). Heffner et al. (2010) noted some measures, as in the case with Chronic Obstructive Pulmonary Disease (COPD), were fragmented and had no impact on the quality of care in terms of effectiveness or efficiency because of other underlying issues such as patient characteristics or employee commitment to the quality measurement.

Quality measures that focus on only one specific area cannot produce holistic change. Werner and McNutt (2009) argued, even if specific quality measures are implemented, those quality measures provided improvement only for a specific area of clinical care that could vary resulting from organizational context. Werner and McNutt argued no solution to address the factors that contributed to poor quality existed as these factors were varied across organizations. They agreed the focus should not be on measuring quality as a stand-alone effort. Werner and McNutt cautioned that providing perfect quality care was a challenge, and such an effort required continuous attention.

Blumenthal and Kilo (1998) also suggested "survival requires long-term investment and rapid execution of activities that add fundamental value to products and services" (p. 645). A theory of continuous improvement was ideal to achievement of value-based health care quality improvement goals. A focus solely on measures and outcomes did not assess underlying causes that affected the variations and outcomes in quality and, consequently, did not guarantee increased quality of performance.

Value-Based Health Care Framework for Success

A suitable framework to increase the impact of pay-for-performance to achieve more holistic changes of improvement was a collaborative model integrating various processes within an organization. Berwick et al. (2008) advised change would be difficult, resulting from culture, technology, motivation, and demand. Berwick et al. suggested a quality improvement design that recognizes the population (patient) as the center of concern, understands policy constraints through decision-making, and has an integrator who can coordinate the resources of the infrastructure to spearhead efforts to achieve health care goals. Finberg, (2012) and Chodhury, Kapur, Saxena, and Topdjian (2011) concluded various systems of reform needed to be integrated to promote accountability and efficiency in value-based health care and not just focus on one area. These authors emphasized a collaborative model considering delivery of care, payment mechanisms, consumer engagement, and research in care processes and outcomes.

The IOM report, *Crossing the Quality Chasm*, initially provided a framework of four levels of the needed changes for an improved system (Berwick, 2002). The four levels follow:

> *These four levels are the experience of patients (Level A), the functioning of small units of care delivery (Level B), the functioning of the organizations that house or support the micro-system (Level C), and the environment of policy, payment, regulation, accreditation, and other ... factors (Level D) that shape the behavior, interests, and opportunities of the organizations at Level C. (p. 83)*

This framework addresses key areas such as highlighting the value of care, engaging in cost-efficient practices, and developing a commitment of do no harm. It seems Medicare's expectation is the value-based, health-care initiative would provide this framework as it was supposed to improve patient experience, increase the functionality of multiple pockets of care mainly through efficiency, resulting in monetary incentives, changes in organizational behavior to a more patient-centric, and a mindful use of resources mindset.

Total Quality Management and Value-based Care

Because there are several problems associated with the initiative that may affect continued quality sustenance, a more suitable and already validated framework that supports transformation is TQM. The three main principles of TQM of customer satisfaction, continuous improvements in organizational process and employee involvement in quality improvement strategies, which can promote changes greater than a sole focus the outcome measures. Other models also recognize the need for a holistic and integrated approach and share similar structures.

Dahlgaard, Pettersen, and Dahlgaard-Park (2011) summarized the IOM's goals and recommended a "4P" model as framework for building quality and organizational excellence. The model focused on people, partnerships, processes, and products. This holistic approach encouraged change in practices that contributed to underuse, overuse, misuse of resources, and ways to keep the interests of the patient central to improvement strategies. These models are devoid of a framework of specific strategies to guide success in value-based health care.

Little research exists on the IOM's proposed framework. The positive impact of TQM in achievement of quality and sustained business excellence is apparent in the reviewed literature. A theoretical model that could serve as a framework of value-based health care was that of expanding Donabedian's model of structure-process-outcomes to include Deming's broad concept of TQM. Despite the lack of improvement sustenance, the views of these seminal thinkers remain the underlying foundations of the definition of quality to include an increased emphasis on the patient. The theories and principles of Donabedian's model and Deming's concepts could be useful to sustaining success in value-base health care. The Donabedian and Demming concepts provided direction on where to develop and implement, as well as an avenue for use of multiple evidence-based tools for sustaining improvement. Donabedian's concept of process of the delivery of health care aligns with the IOM's goals of health care of delivering safe, effective, and patient-centric care.

A more recent adaptation to Donabedian's model included consumer acceptance and experience dimension to the mode, structure, process, outcome, and patient experience (Sheingold & Leid, 2001). This adaptation was an important dimension as it directly related to the HCAPS portion (the eight non-clinical measures) of value-based health care. The goal of efficiency was not explicitly addressed within Donabedian's model, but is achievable using Deming's TQM principles. Although process and outcome measures were more popular, the foundation of Deming's TQM principles were better suited to guide actions to increase quality in organizational activities/characteristics. According to

Sadikoglu (2008), the goals of TQM are to help organizations improve their customer satisfaction, products, and service to maximize profitability.

During the first part of the 21st Century, researchers shared similar constructs for TQM. These constructs were top-management support (or leadership), customer focus, supplier relationship, and employee involvement (Sadikoglu (2008). Authors presented between 5-20 factors essential to facilitating performance excellence. These factors embodied organizational behavior, that when practiced in unison, would support each other and result in increased performance through customer satisfaction, better outcomes, and increased efficiency. A universal agreement did not exist to identify the best factors. Some authors chastised each other for omitting important factors, concentrating on unimportant areas, and/or emphasized more factors than necessary. These factors include leadership, strategic planning, training, developing, process management, knowledge, employee involvement, communication, measurement, analysis, feedback, customer satisfaction, product design, benchmarking, supplier management, and organizational culture (Flynn et al., 1995; Fotopoulos & Psomas, 2009; Khamalah & Lingaraj, 2007; Leape et al., 2009; Lenka & Suar, 2008; Mahapatra & Khan, 2006; Mohammad, Mann, Grigg, & Wagner, 2011; Porter & Parker, 1993; Yusuf, Gunasekaran, & Dan, 2007).

After a comprehensive synthesis of available literature, Tralib and Rahman (2010) presented nine factors that promoted quality output and sustained excellence. These factors included "top-management commitment, customer focus, training and education, continuous improvement and innovation, supplier quality management, employee involvement, employee encouragement, benchmarking, quality information, and performance measurement" (Tralib & Rahman, 2010, p. 370). Inclusion of output and sustained factors into a framework to help leaders organize their business strategies may foster sustained quality in the health-care organization's clinical processes.

Total Quality Management and Business Performance

The practice of TQM strategies was effective in addressing structural and process activities that directly and indirectly influenced patient and organizational outcomes. Empirical evidence existed to suggest strategies geared toward these non-clinical structural and process activities led to improved business performance as indicated by increased efficiency and effectiveness of services and products, which ultimately resulted in improved financial performance (Sila, 2007; Yaacob, 2010). These non-clinical strategies tested and benefited many industries including manufacturing, automobile, and health care. Proponents of TQM practices reiterated the need for leadership to provide oversight to improvement efforts. Under the guidance of leaders, the workforce understood and coped with changes in the expectations as well as being equipped to deliver services that exceeded expectations. Blumenthal and Kilo (1998) suggested, "Survival requires long-term investment and rapid execution of activities that add fundamental value to products and services" (p. 645). A theory of continuous improvement may be ideal to achieving the goals of the newest method of health-care reform.

Quality Improvement Tool for Success

The framework of TQM serves to provide leaders a structural understanding of non-clinical factors on processes and outcomes; leaders need a tool to guide actions to achieving the best possible outcomes. Not only is this framework important to financial sustainability, it is important for national health-care reform goals. Quality improvement is demanding, especially with an added burden of reimbursements being withheld if Medicare pay-for-performance outcomes are unmet. Studies showed, that with successful implementation, organizations will experience improvement in services or products, customer satisfaction, and in financial performance. Total Quality Management (TQM) was one of the most recognized model and was a framework that encompassed non-clinical and clinical factors that could be put into practice with the Baldrige model. The Malcolm Baldrige model continued to provide results and sustained excellence (Evans & Jack, 2003). Curkovic, Melnyk, Calantone, and Handfield (2000) concluded the criteria of the Malcolm Baldrige Criteria for Performance Excellence model exemplified TQM core principles.

    With achieving performance outcomes in value-based care, the challenge was not knowing which approach is appropriate or would be best suited for the organization. A framework of total quality management may help organizations achieve desired results. The framework will prevent health-care leader from wasting resources on strategies they assumed will work or possibly ignoring other aspects of care that could affect quality outcomes. Using a tool generalizable to all organizations is an approach to improving quality within the health-care industry. To alleviate the burden of not having any real framework from the value based model, leaders could use a tool such as the Malcolm Baldrige Criteria for Performance Excellence that increased the probability for success. A major benefit of using this renowned model, and experiencing success, is that it would encourage organizations to repeat quality assurance efforts and to maintain superior levels of clinical quality and consequently business excellence.

Malcolm Baldrige Criteria for Performance Excellence as a Tool for Success

The Malcolm Baldrige Model for Performance Excellence was a tool used to practice the elements of Total Quality Management (TQM) and promote sustained continuous improvement through collaborative efforts rather than a focus on clinical outcomes. The Malcolm Baldrige Criteria for Performance Excellence model exemplified TQM core principles (Curkovic et al., 2000; Hellsten & Klefsjö, 2000). The Baldrige model used in value-based, health care could benefit patients and organizations, as well as sustain quality in the industry. This useful tool integrated a range of organizational strategies beyond those that focused solely on outcomes. The model's approach allowed leaders to evaluate the entire healthcare business system, that is ... the structure, processes to develop strategic plans to ensure the care delivered (rooted in value), and the system sustained would ensure continuous improvement. Use of a tool generalizable to all organizations was an approach to accelerating quality improvement efforts regardless of whether the organization was already performing well or struggling.

Malcolm Baldrige Performance Excellence Model

In 1987, to stimulate an increase in the performance, productivity, and the competitive position of United States' business, President Ronald Regan implemented the Malcolm Baldrige National Quality Improvement Act. The award was used to recognize the quality efforts and improvements in organizations in the United States. Malcolm Baldrige, the Secretary of Commerce, whom the award was named after, had developed a set of criteria based on TQM strategies. These strategies provided business leaders with a tool to assess operations, design, and implement strategies for improvement. One of the purposes of the Malcolm Baldrige award was to heighten awareness of quality and increase quality standards. An increase in quality led to sustained business excellence through maintaining the competitive edge and maximizing profitability (NIST, 2010).

The Malcolm Baldrige Award's purpose was to provide an understanding of organizational processes, and to guide and manage strategies for business excellence. The Baldrige approach used a systematic approach to focus on the customer by using various strategies in areas critical to success. Originally designed for manufacturing firms, the award contained criteria specifically for health care, education, and service companies (Prajogo & Brown, 2004). Research proved the applicability in various industries; the model was presumed to be beneficial to ensuring continued and sustained quality improvement efforts in value-based healthcare. The Malcolm Baldrige criteria supported the goals of value-based health care for promotion of positive customer experiences and provided direction to achieve satisfaction.

Another key purpose of the model's criteria essential to the proposed research was it can facilitate identification of other organizations as role models for sharing information on best practices, vital to overall success of value-based health care. Health-care organizations strived to achieve the Malcolm Baldrige award based on the institution's commitment to quality and excellence. It was appropriate to use the Baldrige model as the conceptual framework for this research. Between 2010 and 2013, CMS will require all health-care organizations to participate in a value-based program. Organizations did not need to apply for the award, but could use the Baldrige criteria to guide strategic goals to increase quality outcomes and sustained organizational excellence. The Malcolm Baldrige criteria could drive performance excellence and serve as a suitable comprehensive theoretical tool to facilitate success in Medicare's value-based health care.

Advantages of Malcolm Baldrige Criteria

The values of the Baldrige model, that included the delivery of consistent positive experiences and the ability to act both ethically and strategically, enhanced the goals of value-based health care. The Baldrige criteria tool also facilitated sustained excellence through continued assessment of efforts of what to do to increase effectiveness and capabilities as well as provide insight into areas where gaps in performance occur (Evans & Jack, 2003; NIST, 2013). The Baldrige criteria encouraged leaders with pertinent questions to think and act strategically to align organizational processes with resources and therefore attain sustainable results (NIST, 2013). According to NIST (2013), the Malcolm Baldrige criteria "focus fosters understanding, communication, sharing, alignment, and integration while supporting innovative and diverse approaches" (para. 6). Leader's answers to these questions provide insight to identify areas that need improvement. Malcolm Baldrige criteria questions are not specific and rigid; instead, the questions serve to help organizations identify areas health-care leaders needed to implement strategies for results.

When criteria were used, organizations can gain valuable insight to relationships between processes and results. According to NIST (2013), "the use of the criteria leads to action-oriented cycles of improvement with four stages:

1. Designing and selecting effective processes, methods, and measures (approach)
2. Executing approach with consistency (deployment)
3. Assessing progress and capturing new knowledge, including seeking opportunities for innovation (learning)
4. Revising plans based on assessment findings and organizational performance, harmonizing processes and work-unit operations, and selecting better process and results measures (integration)" (para. 14).

This action-oriented cycle was of significance to health-care organizations that adopted the Baldrige criteria … determining areas needing improvement, as well as the approach most effective, to develop and implement strategies geared toward achieving results. This may increase the health-care organization's probability of earning full Medicare reimbursements for medical services provided to implement strategies that may also contribute to a more efficient and capable health-care system. Although the criteria can be applied to any business organization, leaders can choose strategies based on business and clinical needs, capabilities, and resources.

The Building Blocks of Malcolm Baldrige

The Malcolm Baldrige Criteria for Performance Excellence was based on four basic elements and seven criteria (Kumar, Choisne, de Grosbois, & Kumar, 2009). These four elements were:

- *Driver.* Senior leadership guides the organization to quality improvement and sustained excellence through creation of values, and goals (NIST, 2013).

- *System.* This refers to the strategic processes designed for meeting the organization's quality and performance requirements (NIST, 2013).

- *Measures of progress.* "Measures of progress provide organizational leaders with results, [which guides their actions] to improving customer value and company performance" (NIST, 2013, p. 15).

- *Goal.* The goal of quality improvement strategies is sustaining business excellence and consequently deliver high quality of service and products to customers (NIST, 2013).

The seven criteria of the MNBQA provided leaders with strategic guidance leadership, "strategic planning, customer focus, measurement, analysis and knowledge management, workforce focus, and process management and results" (NIST, 2013, p. iii). The seven criteria embodied the TQM principles and the model could be essential to instituting successful TQM systems.

- *Leadership* addresses efforts by senior leadership to guide the organization in accomplishing the mission and objectives. The category addresses the need for leaders to communicate with staff to share the vision to create a high-performance environment (NIST, 2013).

- *Strategy Development and Implementation* are efforts, which the organization prepares for its future sustenance through short and long-term goals. The category addresses the necessary resources needed to accomplish plans as well as how to adapt plans should circumstances change (NIST, 2013)

- *Customer and Market Focus* efforts, which the organization undertakes to understand its market and meet the expectations of its stakeholders, for example, listening to the voice of its customers (NIST, 2013)

- *Measurement, Analysis, and Knowledge Management* is the collection and analysis of data to improve its performance and efficiency. The category addresses how the organization uses data to align measure and analyze its strategies to ensure optimum performance (NIST, 2013).

- *Workforce Focus* efforts taken by the organization to train, develop, and motivate employees to achieve organization goals (NIST, 2013)

- *Operation Focus* is the organization approach to identify ways to manage operations efficiently and effectively. The focus of this category is on design and implementation of processes to improve their work system, or to create value for its customers and ensure performance excellence (NIST, 2013)

- *Results* are defined as the organization's business practices as reflected by its financial and operational performance, stakeholder satisfaction, social responsibility, and organization sustainability (NIST, 2013).

Malcolm Baldrige Model Criticism

The Malcolm Baldrige model underwent numerous criticisms in the 1990s. Critics touted it was unfair, unethical, superficial, devoid of quality management, and noted as hypocritical; it did not sustain performance excellence (Jacob et al., 2012). These criticisms were of limited merit as the judgments were based on lack of knowledge of the criteria and not understanding the goals of the model.

In terms of creditability in sustaining excellence, Loomba and Johannessen (1997) refuted the claim stating no program is perfect. Loomba and Johannessen stated that focus should not be distracted from the underlying principle of continuous improvement and quality management. Loomba and Johannessen advised the model is not the ultimate set of guidelines for achieving performance excellence; instead the model could be used as a "catalyst to bring revolutionary change, not just to the U.S. business community, but to American society" (1997, p. 60). Although a Baldrige excellence award's prestige may be sought by any organization, the value is in the Baldrige model's contents and process.

Other critics argued the program took time to implement and failure was likely if leaders were not willing to commit time and resources to understand the necessary components of the model (Chrusciel & Field, 2003). Chrusciel and Field found the issue of preventable medical harm remained the same over a six-year period in a study of 10 hospitals in North Carolina. Although these research findings from the North Carolina hospitals cannot be generalized to the rest of the United States, the results of the research study related to these health-care organizations were of concern because these hospitals' initiatives increased patient safety, quality, and effectiveness of the healthcare organization's processes. Landrigan et al. (2010) found, despite implementing various initiatives and allocating resources to address quality issues, the impact of quality improvement efforts remained little-to-modest in effect. Landrigan et al. (2010) could not rule out the impact of smaller quality improvements; nevertheless, the results reflected quality in the organization's systematic improvements were not resulting in a timely manner. The counter argument was the Malcolm Baldridge model had resources to assist organizations with implementation, as well as facilitated sharing of information from those who have already implemented quality improvement strategies. Most recipients of the Malcolm Baldrige award stated it was important to recognize quality improvement as a journey, not a destination, and the feedback received was worth the time and resources expended (Goonan & Muzikowski, 2008).

Validating the Malcolm Baldrige Criteria

Researchers evaluated the Malcolm Baldrige criteria and found the constructs to be valid dimensions that drove quality improvement (DeBaylo, 1999; Evans & Jack, 2003; Flynn & Saladin, 2001; Pannirselvam & Ferguson, 2001; Wilson & Collier, 2000). Research showed the relationship between the concepts in the criteria of the model, increased and improved business operations, products and services which led to increased and sustained customer satisfaction. The Malcolm Baldrige quality criteria is recognized as a valid tool for designing and implementing quality improvement strategies based on business process improvement areas identified through the institution's self-assessment (Foster, Johnson, Nelson, & Batalden, 2007; Young, 2002).

In one qualitative study, Foster et al. (2007) built on earlier research works of Donaldson and Mohr (2000) and Nelson et al. (2003). Donaldson, Mohr, and Nelson et al. sought to identify the characteristics of clinical practices and procedures within micro-systems that provided high quality and cost-efficient care. Foster et al. (2007) collected data from 20 high-performing, micro-systems through personal interviews leadership, medical staff, and financial records with the intent of determining any correlation to identify if the Malcolm Baldrige criteria could account for success characteristics of these high performing clinical systems. The micro-systems consisted of a small group of people who provided health care to individuals through clinical and business aims linked to specific processes. Foster et al.'s results identified the micro-systems' success characteristics were supported by the Malcolm Baldrige model in the categories of leadership, staff focus, performance results, process improvement, and information technology. The concept of high-performance micro-systems correlated with the Baldrige model despite the researchers not specifically focusing on the Malcolm Baldrige assessment model during the interview, but through an analysis of the answers, according to the Malcolm Baldrige model criteria. Foster et al. validated the Malcolm Baldrige model as a robust model organizations could use to better understand the organization's system, in which corrective focus should occur (e.g., staff, processes, patient), and business process, and medical procedures areas to improve through productivity, efficiency, and outcomes via an analysis of quality performance.

Jayamaha et al. (2008) found the constructs of the Baldrige criteria were valid. Jayamaha et al.'s results, collected from 91 organizations in New Zealand, showed the constructs influenced each other to some degree (some more than others), to produce satisfactory business results. Fening, Pesakovic, and Amaria (2008) confirmed a positive relationship between each of the constructs within the criteria and performance indicators, such as profitability, customer satisfaction, and growth in their study of 116 businesses in Ghana. Studies by Stephens, Evans, and Matthews (2005), Nielsen (2005), Williams (2004), and Bell and Elkins (2004) demonstrated the MBNQA criteria positively affect quality improvement in organizations and leads to sustained performance. These studies justified the Malcolm Baldrige criteria as guidelines to improve organizational performance.

A 2000 study, conducted by Wilson and Collier, provided results validating the Malcolm Baldrige criteria as consistent best predictors of performance excellence in organizations. Wilson and Collier's study supported the Malcolm Baldrige theory that leadership drives results and causal relationships between the criteria were significant in producing positive financial results. Wilson and Collier's study findings confirmed the general theory that each category within the Malcolm Baldrige criteria influenced the impact of the other. Badri et al. also supported this relationship between the constructs in the 2006 study. Leadership drives organization excellence wherein both (leadership and organization) have an impact on business and customer results.

Chapter Summary

The health-care industry needs quality and cost reform. Quality improvement gurus have proposed concepts to address issues of poor quality clinical and business practices within health-care systems and that of poor health care delivered to patients. The literature review found despite many improvement challenging health-care organizations for strategies and ideas generated, none outside the Malcolm Baldridge criteria sustained levels of quality needed to maintain an efficient and effective system. Medicare officials proposed a pecuniary motivation would bring about necessary clinical quality improvements. Reimbursement from traditional fee-for-service to one based on value of health-care deliverables had significant implications for the future of health care. Although research in business strategies of value-based health care was new, the keys to success should be focused on a systemic approach to understand the root causes of poor clinical outcomes and design improvements around this business process knowledge, while keeping the patient at the center of primary efforts. Value-based health care has potential to reform general health care through cost reductions, more efficient processes, and emphasizing the quality value of care. This value-based theory concept lacks a holistic framework to realize the potential of the reimbursement and quality initiative.

The literature review revealed a focus on outcomes and performance measures may not provide the continued levels of quality performance intended by Medicare officials. Critics argued use of performance outcomes as sole indicator for quality performance is not sufficient to bring about the necessary changes within the health-care system. A discussion of the advantage of using TQM as the framework to promote success of Medicare's value-based health care initiative goals was presented in this chapter. The research supported improvements in business dimensions of an organization that synergistically promoted increased quality, reduced costs, and valued results-based outcomes to the patient. This concept was important to maintain financial sustainability, but to bring about necessary change in resource utilization in the health-care industry.

The Malcolm Baldrige Criteria for Performance Excellence offered a suitable tool that promoted the principles of TQM and has proven to increase quality output and sustain operations excellence. Use of this tool could aid organizations in development of more refined business strategies to promote success in

Medicare's value-based, health-care initiative. The Malcolm Baldrige criteria integrated non-clinical and clinical factors that could increase quality and value for patients as well as ensure organizations received medical care related invoice reimbursements. The Malcolm Baldrige criteria were non-prescriptive and flexible thus allowed struggling organizations to gain full reimbursements once they identified the quality and financial balance to perform better, and those already performing well to accelerate their quality improvement efforts further.

The adoption and implementation of the Malcolm Baldrige 'quality assurance' criteria can provide health-care organization leaders with the knowledge of business strategies to implement into their respective organizations to ensure the health-care entities sustained quality and financial improvements and necessary clinical results to receive maximum Medicare reimbursement for medical and healthcare services provided. Continued research is important for the financial sustainability of health-care organizations. Continued research could also help determine the financial future state of the health-care industry. As the Baldridge criteria focuses on value delivered to its customers and sustained operational excellence, the use of the Malcolm Baldrige tool will aid organizations to fulfilling national health care goals of improving the health-care system – one that is safe, delivers health care rooted in value that improves the quality of life for patients, and avoids unnecessary waste.

Chapter 3

Methodology

An exploratory, qualitative methodology allowed an investigation of the best business practices that health-care leaders find important to ensure effectiveness, efficiency, and delivery of high quality services and health care rooted in value. Through an exploration of practices, this research study provided health-care leaders a guide to the business strategies that could aid in providing the quality health care expected: accountability in health care practice, services, and maintenance of the health-care organization's financial viability through efficiency.

The research study's questions established the foundation and methodology for the study. The main research question required an understanding of participants' perspectives and experiences with strategies that promoted improvement in efficiency, increased accountability, and enhancement of the value of care delivered.

The sub-question sought to determine how leaders maintained a balance between the organization's quality and financial goals. The research question and sub-question investigated were as follows:

RQ1: What are the best business strategies health-care leaders use to increase the value of care for success in Medicare's value-based health care program?

a. How do organizations sustain the balance between increasing the value of care, lowering costs, and sustaining their financial growth?

Research Design

Research on business strategies of value-based health care was a relatively new concept. Lowder (2009) discussed the importance of choosing a method that met demands of a research study and supported research. In determining an approach most appropriate for this research study, the research required the methodology's ability to be fluid, exploratory, and to understand business practices adding value to quality of care and to maintain organizational financial viability. An exploratory, qualitative case study, research design was chosen to explore business practices leaders deemed most suited for value-based health care and strategies used to maintain a quality-financial alignment. An exploratory design allowed discovery of phenomena of value-based health care (Cooper & Schlinder, 2011).

Qualitative Design Suitability

A qualitative research design was more suitable for several reasons. First, since this research study was a qualitative study, the researcher was directly involved in data collection, being present in interviews as opposed to detached in an anonymous survey. Second, the research context was of key importance to the health-care industry. Yin (2003) emphasized an understanding of the context of the participants and their environment was critical because it enabled the researcher to explore the significance and the impact of the phenomena. The research context was of key importance in describing the outcomes, as the research environment may have influenced heavily the type of business practices implemented. A qualitative methodology allowed the researcher to study the people, processes, and events in a unified manner in their natural setting (Miles & Huberman, 1994; Reason & Rowan, 1981). Third, data analysis emerged from the qualitative data; that is, analysis was more inductive versus trying to determine a cause and effect relationship as with a quantitative approach (Cooper, Reeves, & Levinson, 2008). This qualitative research design also allowed the researcher to be creative and innovative in presenting descriptive results to the intended audience. The multiple perspectives obtained through data collection helped the researcher deliver a description-thick interpretation, for a richer summary of data.

Quantitative versus Qualitative

Much of the seminal review took a quantitative approach. Quantitative research used specific and controlled standards, as well as statistical analysis to test, justify hypotheses, and account for the relationships between the variables in question (Corbin & Strauss, 2007). Proponents of quantitative research argue that qualitative research is *unscientific* and does not generate hard evidence (Denzin & Lincoln, 2005). Researchers viewed quantitative research as *the gold standard* for conducting research (Robson, 2002). It was not until the 1970s that sociologists and anthropologists introduced qualitative methods to the health care field (Cohen & Crabtree, 2008). Researchers argued, that to understand the problems that occur in everyday life, the use of the (quantitative) *gold standard* was not always practical (Robson, 2002). A quantitative methodology was not always reasonable, because humans behave in unpredictable ways. Rigid and controlled methods were not useful for studying such social behavior (Creswell, 2009; Riege, 2003; Robson, 2002). Although it is possible to use statistical models to assess the success of quality goals proposed by Medicare, a qualitative methodology enabled the researcher to explore 'how' leaders examined and dealt with the issues of quality improvement.

Characteristics of a qualitative methodology allowed the researcher to assimilate the numerous factors that underlie value-based health care from multiple perspectives. Key characteristics of a qualitative study were its lack of dependency on numerical data to gain knowledge, and its focus on the human element to discover an explanation of the subject (Creswell, 2009). Creswell discussed that qualitative research provided a more thorough understanding of the participants as compared to the sole use of statistical models. Qualitative design allowed the researcher to explore strategies that affected the business success of value-based health care. Data obtained through multiple participants' responses and published organizational documents served as one of the units of analyses to explore the topic of value-based, health care. As a result of the qualitative research and methodology focusing on these characteristics, this method provided the researcher an opportunity to fully describe each participant's experiences and gain detailed information of the presumed best business strategies, that work to achieve alignment of business operations and health care goals.

Advantages of Qualitative Methodology

A qualitative methodology provided the opportunity to probe participants to help further explore the topic and gain insight to participant's experiences. As value-based health care is influenced by many factors and is not a static phenomenon, such a methodology allowed the researcher an opportunity to describe fully each participant's experiences and gain detailed information of the best implemented business strategies that worked to achieve profitable alignment of business processes and health-care clinical goals. Different factors influence health-care outcomes. A qualitative methodology, according to Pope and Mays (2008), and Gall, Borg, and Gall (2002), facilitated studying persons in natural settings and allows interaction in their study participants' own language and terms. It was appropriate to choose this qualitative method of inquiry that was flexible, as well as permitted discovery and interpretation of a specific problem.

A qualitative research design was advantageous as it studied persons in natural workplace settings and allowed interaction in their own language and terms (Pope & Mays, 2008). Qualitative research is directed through social constructivism and is concerned with interpreting the behavior of individuals while taking into consideration the context in which the phenomenon was occurring (Creswell, 2009; Gall et al., 2009; Patton, 2002). By using a qualitative research design, the goal was to generate an in-depth description of the business strategies organizations used to support value-based health care to achieve CMS's health care quality goals and maintain organizational financial viability.

Case Study

A case study approach was one of the qualitative research designs available. Creswell (2009) identified five approaches to qualitative research: narrative research, phenomenology, grounded theory, ethnography, heuristic, and case study. These five approaches shared several characteristics including stressing the importance of the participant's frame of reference, conducting research in the participant's natural environment, interpretation of data as collected, and use of rich, thick descriptions in sharing the participants' discoveries (Creswell, 2009). A case study could explore a variety of topics in any setting. A case study could be performed on a group, institution, geographic region, or within an identified time-period. The study could be as simple as studying only one individual or as complex as involving an analysis of multiple cases (Creswell, 2009; Gangeness & Yurkovich, 2006; Nelson & Quintana, 2005). A case study was deemed the most suitable method for answering the research questions and presented substantial and multi-faceted details of the phenomenon of value-based health care, primarily for its advantages of using multiple data collection methods, the methodology's flexibility, and in facilitating an in-depth exploration of successful business strategies of value-based, health care.

A case study's purpose was to advance knowledge about human beings and their interactions in their environment. The case study approach facilitated this researcher's exploration of causal links for business practices most effective in supporting value-based health care. Case studies could be used for several purposes such as providing description(s), testing a theory, generating new theories, developing knowledge through an exploration, and a detailed and thorough analysis of the issue (Creswell, 2009; Baxter & Jack, 2008; Eisenhardt, 1989; Robson, 2002; Wilding & Whiteford, 2005). A case-study approach also allowed description(s) of the context in which these practices were most effective, and possibly provide description for factors or situations that contributed to increased success in maintaining the quality-financial balance. Yin (2009) discussed that a qualitative research study methodology allowed, "… an empirical inquiry that investigates a contemporary phenomenon within its real-life context, especially when the boundaries between phenomenon and context are not … evident" (p. 18). Yin offered that case studies were flexible and could adapt to the context of the research situation. The study of best business practices, that supported value-based health care, originated from the perspective of health-care personnel involved in quality improvement whom could share experiences with improving efficiency, added value to the delivery of care, and increased accountability in services and processes. Use of a case study approach permitted the necessary exploration, description, and explanation of the value-based health care in different organizations.

Unit of Analysis

In this single case study, participants were chosen as the unit of analysis. It was assumed that, understanding the participants' perspectives of the changing culture in health care and experiences with practices that provided the best outcomes in terms of value and cost for the organization, would increase success in participation in the value-based purchasing program within Medicare. An exploration of the participants via thorough data collection provided a deeper insight and helped capture evidence to deliver a rich description of the strategies used (Creswell, 2009; Gibbert, Ruigrok, & Wicki, 2008; Ridder, Hoon, & McCandless, 2009). This description could be beneficial to health-care organization and clinical business leaders, especially those not yet participating in Medicare value-based program. Also, consistent with the case study approach, was collection of data through various methods. The primary data source obtained through participant interviews was triangulated through analysis of printed quality reports available to the public from the organization's website as well as national, quality websites.

Fellow researchers considered the research design and outcomes in case-study research to be valid if the studies showed credibility, conformability, transferability, and dependability. To ensure those four criteria were met, the researcher followed the processes of a qualitative case study, similar to authors Creswell recommended. This process involved adequately identifying suitable organizations, using quotes effectively, providing a description the reader could understand, and ensuring bias was minimized (Stake, 1995).

Summary

Of the qualitative methodologies reviewed to include narrative, ethnographic, phenomenological, and grounded theory; a single case study was deemed the most suited method for answering the research questions and presenting substantial and multifaceted details of the phenomenon of value-based health care. The study's intent was not to tell a detailed story, develop a theory, or understand lived experiences of a phenomenon. The study's intent was specific to explore the issue of value-based health care in local health organizations and was bounded by this topic. Consequently, a case study approach was deemed most suitable for this research. A single case study was appropriate because the researcher anticipated these participants had shared similar goals in finding the necessary balance between financial viability and delivering a high quality of care as directed by CMS. Experiences offered unique perspectives of the phenomenon under this research study.

Population

The targeted population for this exploratory case study was health-care professionals, both male and female, who were either members of American College of Healthcare Executives, the Institute of Health Improvement, the National Association for Healthcare Quality, Association of Healthcare Executives, Institute of Healthcare, Healthcare Management, The American Society for Quality, Baldrige Quest for Excellence, Healthcare Executive Network, Healthcare Financial Management Association, Medical Imaging Network, or the National Association for Healthcare Quality. These noted organizations have thousands of members who were potentially eligible for participation. The listed associations and groups provided a forum for open discussion by its participants via a professional network website, LinkedIn.com. This social website, founded in 2002, had a network of 200 million members in 2013 (LinkedIn.com, 2013). This diverse group of business-professional individuals comes from a variety of organizations in terms of location, size, and ownership.

Sample Framework

This research study employed purposeful sampling to recruit participants. Creswell (2009) suggested sampling those who can provide various perspectives of the problem under investigation. Sampling is choosing the most suitable representation of the population to make a generalization of the whole population (Goulding, 2005). The sample framework used for this exploratory case study was health-care professionals who served in a leadership role (director or manager) with experience in quality improvement.

Purposeful sampling involved choosing subjects who were exemplars of the phenomenon and possessed the most relevant information to help the researcher learn a substantial amount of the topic and answer the research questions (Creswell, 2007; Patton, 2002; Polkinghorne, 2005). Because the goal was to understand the experience, sampling could not be random. Purposeful sampling was recommended for qualitative case study research and was well suited for case study researchers as it was necessary to choose participants considered as information-rich sources to gain the information needed to perform an intensive analysis (Creswell, 2007; Miles & Huberman, 1994). Information-rich cases provided this study's researcher insight on key issues important to the purpose of the inquiry. Studying information-rich participants offered this study's researcher industry insights and an in-depth understanding of the value-based health care and strategies that helped maintain the quality-financial alignment.

Sample

For this study, purposive sampling of 30 participants, male and female health-care professionals who served in leadership roles, and had quality improvement experience, comprised the sample group. The inclusion criteria limited the study to individuals from health-care organizations involved in quality improvement programs operating in the United States. The sample excluded health-care professionals outside the United States, as well as those who had no experience with initiatives to increase quality of care for patients. Participants did not need experience with Malcolm Baldrige criteria, nor did they need to have a specific number of years of experience, in their role in quality improvement.

The case study sample frame also consisted of secondary source of data for content analysis and triangulation. Documents included financial records published since 2012, to help in evaluating themes in organizational business practices in areas of quality and costs. The documents collected from the organization's websites, online databases such as Hospital Compare, Leap Frog, and health care journals added further insight to the issue investigated.

Recruiting Participants

Recruitment of participants occurred in person, via e-mail, telephone introduction, or via a discussion on LinkedIn health care group forum. A letter was sent to potential participants inviting them to share their experiences of quality improvement as it pertained to value-based health care through a personal or telephone interview. The letter included a description and purpose of the research, an informed consent form to ensure participants of their physical and mental rights of protection and privacy, and rights as a participant. Persons interested in participating in the study contacted the researcher via email or telephone from information provided in the letter. After potential participants agreed to share their experiences, the demographic questionnaire, an informed consent form, and the interview questions were sent.

To satisfy the requirements of this qualitative study, along with the university guidelines, availability of participants, time constraints, the expected differences in outcome, and theoretical saturation; the sample population recruited for the case study was 30 participants. This number of participants was chosen in the event the targeted population of at least 20 was not obtained. Should 30 participants have agreed to participant in the study, the researcher would have selected between 20-25 participants based on the greater number of years in quality improvement.

Sample Size

Thirty health-care leaders were selected randomly as participants for this study. Time constraints, the number of participants available, the phenomenon under study, and theoretical saturation were factors that influenced selection of an appropriate sample size (Marshall, 1996). A sample size of 30, although small, was sufficient to gather ample data. Merriam (1998) stated, "The number of participants to sample depends on factors such as questions asked, data gathered, analysis, and resources to support the study" (p. 64). A sample size of 30 was appropriate to enable valid inferences based on the surveyed population. A larger sample may not necessarily provide more information or data might have become redundant if a larger sample was used (Mason, 2010). There was no clear answer for a set number of participants in qualitative studies.

Merriam used Lincoln and Guba's (1985) suggestion that sampling should continue until a point of saturation. The researcher expected, as health-care leaders work simultaneously to achieve national health care goals, the health-care leaders would have shared similar goals and therefore shared similar experiences. Responses among participants, as expected, were consistent and theoretical saturation occurred relatively quickly. Guest, Bunce, and Johnson (2006) found the idea of saturation provides limited guidance for determining sample size. In Guest's et al. literature research, they found limited researchers offering guidelines to determine sample size. Of those found, the sample size ranged from five to 50. Green and Thorogood (2009) also suggested most qualitative researchers found little (identifiable) new research was collected after interviewing roughly 20 people. Ultimately, the research questions determined the optimum number for the size of the sample.

Instrumentation

In this exploratory study, data was collected through interviews conducted by the researcher; the researcher acted as the research instrument of data collection. The role of research instrument (as the interviewer) involved asking pertinent questions relevant to the study and active listening to gain a comprehensive understanding of the participants' answers. This helped to assimilate the large amount of information collected, captured the mood, enabled understanding of important interview concepts, and reduced the need for reading between the lines (Yin, 2009). Active listening was key to representing the context of what was being said. As there was no set protocol for designing, collecting, and analyzing data, the researcher (as the instrument) must be tolerant of ambiguity. The researcher was expected to exercise patience in following leads, listening to answers to research questions, and piecing research information together. As the data collection instrument, it was necessary to maintain sensitivity to the environment, the participants, and the information gathered. Sensitivity reduced bias, especially as contradictory information arose (Yin, 2009). Sensitivity during the interview helped the interviewer realize when to pause for silence, probe further, and/or change the direction of the interview.

Researcher Background and Experience

The researcher's background included conducting job interviews and analyzing scholarly articles. This experience provided some insight into how to conduct the interviews … knowing when to listen and watching for signals to probe for further questioning. The didactic experience to read, critique, and analyze documents helped evaluate public quality improvement documents gathered. Although the researcher had previous experience in interviewing, it occurred in a different setting, and as such, the researcher required additional training in these methods. As far as interviewing is concerned, the key to obtaining good data was to practice interviewing skills. Therefore, to become more competent and knowledgeable on the process, improving interview skills involved role playing with colleagues to have an idea of the time needed for participants to answer questions. The role-playing increased the researcher's sensitivity to respondent's answers to notice cues open for further elaboration or that required the participant to be steered back to on topic (Bryman, 2008). The sessions were recorded for self-evaluation. Observing experienced interviewers via television and the Internet increased the researcher's proficiency and prepared the researcher before the actual interview process. This not only improved the skills, but also built confidence (Merriam, 1998). These interview improvement exercises increased the researcher's capability for conducting effective interviews and compiling data for analysis.

Data Collection

The strength of this case study lies in the ability to explore the topic of value-based health care through documentation, interviews, observation, and physical artifacts as data collection methods (Yin, 2003). The goal of data collection in qualitative research is to obtain information on the essence of personal experiences (Polkinghorne, 2005). The researcher must continuously peel back the surface impressions to capture the pertinent data. It was an iterative process, as data was continuously collected and analyzed simultaneously. Consequently, the main data collection instrument was use of a semi-structured interview that collected data based on the Malcolm Baldrige seven performance excellence criteria.

The participant interview was an appropriate data collection method for this research study as it helped explore participants' experiences with value-based health care and quality improvement business strategies. Hancock and Algozzine (2006) postulated interviews were a common data collection method in case study research. The appropriateness of the data collection method was determined by the researcher's theoretical orientation, the problem, the purpose, and by the sample selected (Merriam, 1998). To obtain relevant data and insight for this study, interviews of the appropriate personnel involved in quality improvement business strategy and collecting public data in related areas were justified, especially since multiple data collection methods were essential to qualitative case studies.

Interviews provided an opportunity to ask specific questions pertaining to various facets of performance excellence and quality improvement, and consequently understand how management interpreted increasing value to develop appropriate business strategies to promote sustenance. The interviews allowed the researcher to attain an in-depth and comprehensive account of personalized information. As quality improvement and value-based health care can have varied meanings, using interviews as the data collection method helped to pool these broad ranges of ideas into recurring themes that may serve as a guideline for new participants or those struggling to maintain their financial-quality alignment.

Data collection began with a recruitment letter via e-mail to the participants to inform them of the study's purpose and request their participation. Thirty participants were contacted and 21 responded. A greater number of participants were contacted in case some participants could not commit time or preferred not to participate. If all 30 participants agreed, the ones with greatest number of years of experience in quality management would have been chosen.

Once participants agreed, and necessary consents obtained, a telephone or face-to-face appointment was set. The participants received a copy of the research study's interview questions and informed consent one week in advance to provide enough time for review. A reminder e-mail issued mid-week served to remind participants of upcoming interview in addition to completing the consent form. The interviews were limited to 30 minutes. All participants were reminded of confidentiality and anonymity. All participants were asked to give their consent, again, prior to the interview. An interview guide helped the interviewee use the allotted time effectively. The researcher also requested verbal consent for recording the interview. All the interviews were recorded using a digital voice recorder to ensure accuracy in collecting the data and to analyze emerging themes later. Of the 21 participants queried, 19 participated via a telephone interview, and two provided answers to the interview questionnaire in written format. The researcher took notes of tone, posture (in person interviews), and remarks that needed further clarification were addressed at the end of the interview. All transcriptions were sent to participants to verify data and clarify any additional questions.

In addition to the interview, the researcher selected text in publicly available documents as part of data collection. This study sought publicly available documents that included public financial records, organizational executive summaries, standard operating procedures, strategic development documents, and quality reports published since 2007. Patton (2002) discussed that documents could provide data about events that occurred before the research started, as well as other things that an interview cannot capture. Choice of two data collection instruments (interviews and reports) helped present a richer description of value-based health care. By using several different data sources, case study researchers were equipped with a wide array of information with the hope of understanding the underlying principles behind the issue (Eisenhardt, 1989).

Publically documents not only added sources of information, but also were used to compare data to determine consistency in the research's findings. Public data was collected from five quality-based organizations' websites, as well as top-performing, health-care organizations, which allowed the researcher to explore patterns in quality improvement initiatives, quality of care, and the influence on financial performance over time. These documents retrieved were from online databases such as Hospital Compare, LeapFrog, the participant's organization's website, and quality-improvement documents provided valuable information about organizational commitment, success, and plans for continued improvement in the delivery of quality health care while reducing overall organizational costs. The content of these documents underwent analysis as it pertained to the Malcolm Baldrige framework. The use of multiple-data collections assisted in accomplishing the goal of the research. The research objective was to obtain enough quality-related, detailed information from each participant who could guide others, especially those not yet participating in Medicare's value based program, The Malcolm Baldrige criteria was publically available from the NIST website. The interview questions could be found in Appendix B.

This case study used an interview guide modeled after the Malcolm Baldrige Criteria for Performance Excellence. The interview instrument used questions adapted from the renowned Malcolm Baldrige Criteria for Performance Excellence model used by organizations in health care and in other industries. This model provided leaders with a systematic perspective for understanding the impact of various elements within the organization on performance. Officials at NIST validated and tested the approach as a reliable tool to leading-edge management practices against which an organization can measure itself in its improvement journey to achieve higher levels of excellence. These criteria provided a valid and reliable framework to help organizations plan a path to performance excellence and to measure improvement(s).

The interview instrument was established using the seven categories the model provided, detailing areas of improvements. Each participant was asked 33 questions from an interview guide adapted from the Malcolm Baldrige criteria found in Appendix B. The core concepts of the criteria were built upon seven categories specific to health care: "[a] Leadership, [b] Strategic Planning, [c] Customer and Market Focus, [d] Measurement, Analysis, Knowledge Management, [e] Workforce Focus, [f] Operation Focus, and [g] Results" (NIST, 2013, p. iii). The interview questions used the criteria to gain a better understanding of the business practices that contributed to success in value-based health care.

Field Test

A field test conducted before actual interviews provided the researcher an opportunity to ensure the interview questions would elicit appropriate answers to the research study's questions. A field test was performed using three personnel who fit the sampling criteria. Field testing the interview questions ensured the interview questions were clear to the participants, did not cause misinterpretation, and elicited responses appropriate to the research question. The field test helped the researcher to note personal behaviors or questions that caused discomfort to the participants or did not convey the intended meaning behind the question. The main intent of engaging these individuals in the field test was to critique the study's interview questions. The results of the interview questions were analyzed to test the feasibility of the analysis approach. Adjustments made included clarifying all questions were based on value-based health care, and one question was restructured to elicit a richer response. The field test also provided the opportunity to fine-tune interview skills or behavior. Another goal of the field testing was to test the functionality of equipment, the process, and the researcher's interview and note-taking skills to facilitate a smoother and more effective interview process.

Data Preparation

The main purpose for data collection was to understand the business practices that facilitated financial success in Medicare's value-based care, as well as to understand how health-care organizations achieve targeted-quality finance balance. The key elements in analyzing qualitative data were reducing the amount of data into manageable pieces (achieved through coding), identifying patterns, creating categories, and then finally presenting them within a framework to be accurately communicated to the reader (Goulding, 2005; Osborne, 1994).

Data preparation began with transcribing interviews from the digital recorder. After transcribing, the audio was replayed to ensure transcription accuracy. A master list of participants with an arbitrary identifier was created and each transcript was given a numerical identifier that matched the list. The master list was secured in a locked drawer. The researcher worked with the anonymized data for the remainder of the study.

Data Analysis

Data analysis for this exploratory case study was guided by the categories of the Baldrige Criteria for Performance Excellence. After each interview was transcribed, all data was sorted by question in each category and placed in tabular form in a Word® document to allow easier analysis and interpretation. Separation of data into each category allowed for a clearer understanding of data collected from all participants. The transcribed data was assessed for bias by taking note of the tone of the data, looking for incomplete representations of the participant's perspective, and any personal comments. For any bias noted, side notes were placed along with the transcription and included with the presentation of data. Merriam (1998) stated it was beneficial to keep track of thoughts, speculations, or hunches during this process.

The researcher read each transcript several times to make sense of these data and identify similar themes using inductive analysis. Inductive analysis, according to Denzin and Lincoln (1998) and Creswell (2007) focuses on like patterns in data. This was done for all questions for each participant. Following this, the interview data was categorized by question and answer so all the answers for one question were placed in one document. This manner of organization prepared the data for coding. The process of coding involved identifying information about the data, and interpreting the constructs as they related to analysis. Merriam (1998) said coding "is nothing more than assigning some form of shorthand designation to various aspects of your data so that you can easily retire specific pieces of data" (p. 164). Coding was accomplished in categories determined by the Malcolm Baldrige performance excellence framework. Use of predefined codes was consistent with the manner Creswell (2007) recommended coding information. Data within each Baldrige category were 'clustered' according to sub-themes that emerged within each predefined code (Miles & Huberman, 1994). The codes were re-reviewed to look for similarity and reduce the number of codes. Upon completion, the researcher reviewed the document for refinement and re-categorized data and emergence of additional themes. Data was reviewed a fourth time to identify patterns in the codes and then regrouped and assigned a descriptor theme to support clustered data. The pre-defined themes and supporting sub-themes were arranged in a tabular matrix to provide a frame of reference in discussion of the findings and conclusions to the research questions.

Coding, developing matrices, and sorting data were very time consuming and subject to human error. To analyze the data, the researcher employed the use of a Computer Assisted Qualitative Data Analysis System (CAQDAS). Qualitative software considered were Atlas.ti, Dedoose, and NVivo. Time constraints to learn new software and availability of knowledgeable personnel, resulted in choosing NVivo, to help organize and make sense of the large amount of data. The use of NVivo helped organize and analyze all the transcribed interviews.

Validity and Reliability

Although this qualitative research study was not concerned with statistical numbers, issues of reliability and validity should be paramount to qualitative researchers when evaluating the overall design and quality of the study (Golafshani, 2003). Findings in case study research are considered valid if they show credibility, conformability, transferability, and dependability wherein that of grounded theory depends upon the credibility of data interpretations (Osborn, 1994; Riege, 2003).

Validity, Johnson (1997) stated, is research that is "plausible, credible, trustworthy and therefore defensible" (p. 282). Validity, from a realist's perspective, refers to the accuracy of a result. Researchers must ensure the relationships established in the findings were true. Maxwell (1992) discussed validity as the authenticity of qualitative research. The main facets of validity include: not distorting the information heard (descriptive validity), the validity of concepts as applied to the phenomena, how concepts were gathered (theoretical validity), and understanding the phenomena from an *emic* rather than *etic* perspective (interpretive validity). Riege (2003) emphasized that avoidance of assumptions or judgments during data collection enhanced the validity of the study.

To ensure this validity of this research, phrases were used close to the participants' accounts, cross checked the information, elicited participant feedback, and engaged reflexivity. The use of these strategies, according to Riege (2003), was to certify the findings were credible, coherent, and an accurate account by the subject (Riege, 2003). The multiple sources of data, proposed in the study, may help reduce bias, and hence increase validity.

Reliability referred to the stability and accuracy of the findings demonstrated when another researcher replicated the process of the case study. To address reliability, the study's methods, data collection, and analysis procedures were explicitly described, so other researchers can re-conduct the study and achieve the exact same results (Riege, 2003). Well documented studies that can be repeated, and achieve the same results, confer reliability of the study (Soy, 1997).

Validity and reliability are key issues for any case study research. Having a high degree of validity and reliability confers confidence in the research design, from data collection to the interpretation of the results and applicability in other settings. The researcher undertook triangulation, member checks, and documenting details to ensure validity.

Ethical Consideration

The ethical consideration for this research study was that no harm occurred to participants during the conduct of the study or in retaliation to the final report of this research. All participants consented to the interview and were made aware of the minimal risks presented by participating in the study. Participants and information gleaned about the participants' representative organizations were guaranteed confidentiality and anonymity. Interviews were numbered to maintain anonymity during the research study. To ensure privacy, a record of actual names was kept in a locked drawer and destroyed after a period of seven years. The data was only accessible only by the researcher. Participants in the research study experienced minimal risk. The study's intent was to describe the optimum healthcare business best practices used by organizations to facilitate success in Medicare, value-based health care; therefore, no possibility of harming participants or the organizations and associations they belong to occurred. Participation was voluntary and participants had the opportunity to ask questions about the nature of the study. A letter code was assigned to each document downloaded from any participants' organization's website. Downloads were kept confidential and maintained on a separate hard-drive, also pass-code protected. The external hard-drive was destroyed along with the interview recordings after a period of seven years as required by Capella University.

Another ethical consideration included avoiding bias and ensuring the researcher's competence to conduct the interview. The researcher remained alert to avoid any personal bias behavior by refraining from any preconceived ideas of the individuals or answers. The researcher made the effort to approach the data with objectivity. Throughout data collection and analysis, a "stance of neutrality" (Patton, 2002, p. 51) was maintained.

The researcher practiced interviewing personnel prior to data collection to ensure proper body language for the few interviews conducted in person, tone of voice and effective use of time. Although the researcher had previous experience in interviewing, it had been a different setting. It was to the researcher's benefit to seek additional training in interviewing methods. The key to obtaining rich data was to practice. The researcher videotaped mock sessions as well as observed and listened to experienced interviewers via television or the Internet to fine-tune interviewing skills. This improved the interview skills, but also built confidence to facilitate successful interview session(s).

Chapter Summary

An overview of the qualitative methodology used in this study to describe the best business practices that facilitated success in Medicare's value-based health care program was provided in this chapter. The population included health-care professional belonging to various executive, financial, quality improvement, and health-care organizations. The participants possessed relevant knowledge to practices best suited to improve the value of care delivered and to achieve maximum reimbursement for medical services provided. Qualitative data collection, using interviews and printed documents, allowed the researcher to obtain a deeper understanding of value-based care using the Malcolm Baldrige Criteria for Performance Excellence. The interviews provided the opportunity for the researcher to encourage participants to share didactic and professional experiences about increasing the value of care for patients while reducing costs. The documentation helped to triangulate data and fill in gaps as needed. A detailed discussion of the research design, sampling, data collection, and data analysis followed. Issues of reliability, validity, in addition to the researcher's experience, and the ethical considerations pertaining to this research were addressed. Chapter 4 presented an analysis of the data collected. A discussion of the results follow in Chapter 5.

Chapter 4

Results

Chapter four presented the findings from analysis of data collected through interviews of 21 health-care professionals. The purpose of this qualitative case study was to explore the best strategies health-care leadership deemed necessary for health-care organizations to operate efficiently and deliver quality services, especially to achieve maximum reimbursement for their services performed. Primary data collection included participants' perspective of strategies that facilitate success in value-based health care. Data was triangulated using publically available documents such as financial reports, organizational executive summaries, standard operating procedures, strategic development documents, and quality reports.

The chapter began with a description of the study and the sample. An explanation of the data collection process and presentation of data follows. Analysis and findings were discussed in the following chapter. The chapter concluded with a summary of the findings.

The Study

In value-based health care, a lack of the best business practices existed that health-care organizations could use to facilitate receiving maximum reimbursement for clinical services provided. Although the clinical goals of value-based health care were clear, it was evident from the literature review that research on the business strategies necessary to implement value-based quality programs in health care was lacking. The focus of previous research studies remained solely on the Medicare clinical measures of quality for specific areas in value-based health care. A possible explanation for the lack of research was the relative newness of the concept. As a result, leaders in health-care organizations leaders must determine the strategies that could produce the best outcomes for both the patient and the organization. Consequently, health-care leaders relied on skills and years of experience to steer the organization's success in achieving quality outcomes and sustaining financial growth.

This study explored the strategies needed to operate efficiently and deliver high quality services rooted in value. Knowledge on these strategies was of significance to organizations, especially to achieve maximum reimbursement for health-care services provided to clientele (patients), reviewed, and submitted to Medicare. An additional purpose of the research study was to investigate how leaders maintained the balance between increasing quality of care, lowering costs, and maintaining organizational financial goals. Patients could benefit from evidence-based strategies and organizations would have a better foundation to attain financial goals. Knowledge in quality and financial arenas was important as the information provided leaders with a guideline of the strategies that promote financial viability and organizational sustainability, rather than guessing the business strategies that could achieve satisfactory outcomes. The outcomes of this qualitative case study could serve as a starting point to help organizational leaders set standards of quality, implement business strategies specific to increase the value of care for patients, reduce unnecessary waste, and promote accountability, effectiveness, and efficiency in health care services and processes.

Research Question and Sub-question

The research question and sub-question for the study were as follows:

Main Research Question 1

What were the best business strategies health-care leaders used to increase the value of care for success in Medicare's value-based health care program?

Sub-question Related to Main Research Question 1

How did organizations sustain the balance between increasing the value of care, lowering costs, and sustaining financial growth?

Description of the Sample

This study involved health-care professionals who have worked in development and implementation of quality improvement strategies. Therefore, a convenience sample of health-care professionals from health-care associations and forums available through the professional network, LinkedIn, and a local network of health-care leaders encompassed the sample frame for this study. The inclusion criteria limited the study to individuals from health-care organizations in the United States who had accepted and provided care for Medicare's patients and were currently or previously involved with a quality improvement program in the research-study participants' health-care organization. This group of individuals (interviewees) came from a variety of health-care organizations in terms of location, size, and ownership. It was neither necessary for participants to have experience with Malcolm Baldrige criteria nor did they need to have a specific number of years in their role in quality improvement.

Health-care professionals, specifically those who served in a variety of functional, clinical areas within quality improvement roles, constituted the sample frame for this study. These professionals were recruited from LinkedIn groups such as American College of Healthcare Executives, the Institute of Health Improvement, The National Association for Healthcare Quality, Association of Healthcare Executives, Institute of Healthcare, Healthcare Management, The American Society for Quality, Baldrige Quest for Excellence, and from a local WA state network of health-care professionals. Recruitment of participants occurred in person, via e-mail, or with a telephone introduction. A letter was sent to potential participants inviting them to share their lived experiences of quality improvement as it pertained to value-based health care through a personal or telephone interview. The letter included a description and purpose of the research and an informed consent to assure participants of their protection and human rights as a participant. Persons interested in the study contacted the researcher via email or from the telephone information provided in the letter. After participants agreed to share their experiences in the study, the demographic questionnaire, an informed consent form, and the interview questions were sent.

To satisfy the requirements of this qualitative study, along with the university guidelines, availability of participants, time constraints, the expected differences in outcome, and theoretical saturation; the sample population recruited for the case study was 30 participants. This number of participants was chosen in the event the targeted population of at least 20 was not obtained. Should 30 participants have agreed to participant in the study, the researcher would have selected between 20-25 participants based on the greatest number of years in quality improvement. Initially, 10 participants responded to the recruitment email. The researcher sent another request and posted another discussion on LinkedIn about the dissertation topic and requesting participants. Six more participants were obtained. In search of more participants, the researcher actively followed-up with potential participants via email and with a telephone call. An additional eight participants were recruited for a total of 24 participants. Of the 24 participants, all but three failed to respond to arrange an interview meeting; therefore, the final sample population was 21 participants.

Prior to the start of the interview questions, participants were reminded again of their human rights as a participant and permission was asked to record the interview session. All participants indicated they understood their rights and agreed for the interview to be recorded. Prior to asking the interview questions, the researcher defined how value-based health care was used for the research. Data collection for this research study included use of a semi-structured interview questionnaire used by the researcher. Each participant was asked 33 questions from an interview guide adapted from the Baldrige criteria found in Appendix B. The core concepts of the criteria were built upon seven categories specific to health care: "[a] Leadership, [b] Strategic Planning, [c] Customer and Market Focus, [d] Measurement, Analysis, Knowledge Management, [e] Workforce Focus, [f] Operation Focus, and [g] Results" (NIST, 2013, p. iii).

Data collection occurred by using a semi-structured, interview questionnaire and lasted between 30 and 45 minutes. Interviews were scheduled for 30 minutes; however, participants were enthusiastic about the topic and provided more detailed answers than expected. Consequently, some participant interviews went beyond the allotted timeframe. Four interviews were conducted face-to-face and 15 interviews were conducted via telephone. Two participants preferred to answer the questionnaire in written format because of scheduling conflicts. All participants were sent a follow-up email to thank them for the participation and to review the transcript for accuracy. More questions, after the interview, were asked if the researcher thought the participants' answers needed additional clarification.

Study Demographic Data

Of the sample, 19% functioned as executive managers, 48% were middle level managers, and 33% functioned as front-line level management leaders. These participants worked in a variety of roles such as chief executive officer, director of clinical operations, consultant, and department managers. Participants' roles included strategy development, implementation, and execution, clinical quality management, business intelligence management, and operations management.

Thirty-eight percent of participants had less than or equal to 10 years of quality management experience whereas 29% had between 11-20 and 21-30 years, and 4% had greater than or equal to 31 years. The sample population consisted of 14% of persons between the ages 30-40, 38% between the ages 41-50, and 48% between the ages 51-60. Gender for this population included 67% males and 33% females. Table 1 presented a summary of the demographic data for study's participants. Appendix B presented the couple of introductory questions from the interview questions that provided brief demographic data.

Table 1 - Study Demographic Data

Age	Number of Participants
30-40	3
41-50	8
51-60	10
Total	21
Gender	
Male	17
Female	7

Age	Number of Participants
Management Level	
Executive	4
Upper	10
Middle	7
Total	21
Years of Quality Management Experience	
≤10	8
11-20	6
21-30	6
≥31	1
Total	21
Years in Current Position	
0-10	19
11-20	1
21-30	1
Total	21

Secondary Data Source

The sample frame consisted of secondary data from publicly available performance reports, organizational executive summaries, strategic development documents, and quality reports of five random health-care organizations in Washington State for 2012/2013. Fifty-three available documents were collected from the organization's websites. Of the documents available, between four and six documents were selected from each organization for a total of 26 documents. This number of documents had sufficient information that closely reflected best practices within the framework of the Baldrige categories. The purpose of this secondary source of information served to triangulate the themes from the responses to the interview questions. Table 2 specifies the category of health-care organization ownership; nonprofit, government-owned, its size, and the number of published documents collected for this research. Organizations with more than 400 employees were considered large organizations for the purpose of this research.

Table 2 - Secondary Data Source Characteristics

Organization	Ownership	Size	Number of Documents
A	Nonprofit	Large	4
B	Nonprofit	Large	5
C	Nonprofit	Large	6
D	Nonprofit	Large	6
E	Government	Large	5
Total			26

Research Methodology Applied
to the Data Analysis

The methodology chosen for this study was an exploratory qualitative inquiry. A qualitative approach was best suited to explore and describe the business strategies health-care leaders use that could facilitate superior performance, organizational effectiveness, and sustain improvement. This method was ideal to capture participants' experiences and was best suited to provide a more thorough understanding of the participants as compared to other models.

Primary Data Analysis

The researcher systematically transcribed participants' responses into appropriate categories of leadership, customer/market focus, workforce focus, operation focus, strategic planning, knowledge / measurement, and results. Responses to the same question were placed in a table. This sorting of data simplified these data for detection of 'like themes' and patterns in each category and was done for each of the seven categories. After this was completed for all the questions, the researcher reviewed the tabular compilation to identify emerging sub-themes for each specific question. Using inductive analysis, thoughts, and concepts were highlighted to identify patterns using inductive analysis (Cooper et al., 2008; Creswell, 2007). Once completed, codes were assigned to these highlighted data. Coding, according to Miles and Huberman (1994), uses a tag that represents a pattern of segments of data. The data were scrutinized several times to ensure codes chosen within each category were appropriate and applicable to the participant's responses and that no new groups of codes were identified (Miles & Huberman, 1994).

The coded transcripts were further scrutinized to similarly clustered codes to further narrow the sub-themes that emerged. Data was reduced further to facilitate easier analysis and synthesis of data because of time constraints and resources dedicated for this study. These sub-themes were placed in a separate Word® document to make triangulation with primary data easier. The majority of data analysis was done manually. The Computer Assisted Qualitative Data Analysis System NVivo was used to assist identifying subthemes from the data.

Secondary Data Analysis

For this study, random health-care organization documents were reviewed for evidence that organizations sought ways to improve the delivery of care and their processes to facilitate a more efficient industry with greater health care outcomes for their patients. Yin (2009) advised to triangulate data as it ensures accuracy of results. Multiple sources of information not only prevent misconception, but they also provide added meaning to data collected (Stake, 2005). Data analysis of secondary data sources increased accuracy and gave added meaning to the primary data collected. Pertinent data points from secondary data were extracted and were placed in the appropriate Malcolm Baldrige category in a similar manner to the primary data. The documents were examined for data specific to the predefined themes reflected by the seven categories of the Malcolm Baldrige criteria. These highlighted data were clustered to organize data according to the emerging sub-themes within the categories. These themes were placed in a separate Word® document to make triangulation with the primary data easier.

Categorical Aggregation of Interview Data

This section contains the analysis of participants' responses to the interview questions that were framed to answer the main research question regarding the business practices that leaders use to facilitate success in value-based health care. A sub-question was developed to gain deeper meaning of these data and understand how health-care leaders integrate their business strategies to maintain a quality-financial alignment. The questions were structured according to the Baldrige Criteria for Performance Excellence categories that consequently established pre-defined themes established for data. Criteria questions were focused on leadership, customer focus, workforce focus, strategy planning, measurement, operation focus, analysis and knowledge, and results.

Themes Identified

Data analysis within the predefined themes identified consistent thoughts. These thoughts were clustered to present sub-themes that emerged. Three to five sub-themes of strategies were discovered within the Malcolm Baldrige framework in this study. Table 3 reflects sub-themes that emerged from predefined main themes.

Table 3 - Themes and Related Sub-themes

Main Theme	Sub-theme 1	Sub-theme 2	Sub-theme 3	Sub-theme 4	Sub-theme 5
Leadership	Quality Defined	Value Defined	Leadership Roles in Value based health care		
Customer / Market Focus	Patient Satisfaction	Patient Engagement	Patient Education		

Main Theme	Sub-theme 1	Sub-theme 2	Sub-theme 3	Sub-theme 4	Sub-theme 5
Work-force Focus	Employee Efficiency	Prevention of Employee Frustration	Workforce Resource Allocation	Training	Incentivizing Behavior
Strategy Planning	Sustainability	Strategy Resource Allocation			
Operation Focus	Optimizing Operations	Preparation for Success			
Measurement, Analysis, and	Data Integration	Measurement Resource Allocation			
Results	Cultural Influence	Measurement of Success	Considerations of Value-Based Health Care		

Presentation of Data and Results

A qualitative methodology guided this exploratory case study. The literature review revealed the Baldrige Criteria for Performance Excellence model exemplified the core principles of TQM (Curkovic et al., 2000; Hellsten & Klefsjö, 2000). The model helped formulate the research and interview questions. The criteria facilitated sustained excellence (Evans & Jack, 2003; NIST, 2013) through an understanding of organizational and a continued assessment of efforts of what to do to increase effectiveness and capabilities as well as provide insight to areas where gaps in performance occur.

Data analysis of the interview data elicited a comprehensive understanding of participants' experience in quality improvement in health care. The responses drawn from the interview questions served as the frame of reference for this study. Data analysis collected identified two to five major sub-themes within each of the pre-defined themes established by the seven categories of the Malcolm Baldrige Criteria for Performance Excellence. Following analysis of the main research question, data were analyzed again and were mapped to the research sub-question.

Research Question and Sub-question

This exploratory qualitative case study analyzed the experiences of 21 health-care leaders and 24 separate organizational documents to answer the main research question, "What are the best business strategies health-care leaders use to increase the value of care delivered for success in

Medicare's value-based health care program?" [and] "How do leaders achieve the balance between increasing the value of care delivered and sustainment of their organizations' financial growth?"

Main Theme 1: Leadership

According to the Malcolm Baldrige criteria, the category of leadership examined how leaders manage and guide their system to performance excellence and sustainability. Leaders communicated and promoted the vision of value and quality to its stakeholders. In terms of value-based health care, Questions 1-7 examined the leaders' defined quality and value and the manner that leaders transformed the culture of the organization from volume-based to one that increases value to its patient. The questions were designed to ascertain how leaders transformed the culture without causing frustration, skills, and behavior necessary for leaders to accomplish such a transformation. Coding and analysis against the leadership category identified multiple definitions of quality and value, and essential roles participants believed leaders should perform to promote success in organizations participating in value-based care.

Quality Defined.

Participants' definition of quality included elements of excellence, safety, and effectiveness and was achieved when outcomes are satisfactory to the patient, or regulatory standards. Participants defined quality primarily from a clinical perspective, that is, the caliber of service delivered to the patient. Participants equated quality as satisfactory through meeting customer expectations, safety through error prevention, defect-free performance through performing tasks correctly, and satisfying clinical outcome requirements. One participant believed it was through an integration of these perspectives that excellence naturally permeated the organization.

Value Defined.

Value-based health care was defined using Medicare's definition prior to the start of each interview as improving the quality/value of care provided for patients at a lower cost (CMS, 2011). When asked, *"What does value based care mean to you?"* (Question 2), it was evident 10 out of 21 participants were not familiar with the interview term value-based health care as a concept other than the researcher's definition. Some participants were aware it was a new reimbursement strategy, whereas others viewed the term solely to increase focus on the patient. Despite the initial concern that participants were not aware of the term, their responses indicated an understanding of underlying precept in value-based health care as a way of improving the care for patients at a lower cost for the benefit of the patient or the organization. Twelve out of 21 participants related value to patient outcomes or that results were worth the resources in which the patient invested, and that patients were satisfied with health care received. In addition to this patient-centric definition of value, nine out of 21 participants believed value meant improvement in operational activities. Value-based efforts, according to participants, included performing duties correctly and finding ways to reduce costs within the organization. None of these nine participants mentioned that improvement in these value-based areas were because of intrinsic motivation or because of regulatory requirements.

Leadership Roles in Value-based Health Care

In response to how leaders transform the culture without causing frustration, and the skills and behavior necessary for leaders to accomplish culture transformation (Questions 3-7), participants voiced their opinion that leaders played a critical role in creating an environment that sustained performance excellence. Participants disclosed it was important for leaders to share the vision and principles of value-based health care. Communication with employees, according to participants, provided a common understanding of the organization's vision, and as such, employees could function effectively and with purpose in their employment roles. Participants believed communication will ultimately transform the health-care organization work-place culture to one that delivers care, rooted in value.

Participants also mentioned leaders have an increased chance of engaging employees in value-based care activities with incentives. Of note, one participant added employees are intrinsically motivated to help patients; therefore, this participant did not stress the need to incentivize employees to perform at their best. Participants shared common beliefs that to transform the culture and promote excellence in value-based health care, leaders should be committed, share decision-making, compassionate, ethical, engaging, and share accomplishments. One participant added that health-care organization leaders should possess additional skills of adaptability and flexibility to deploy the organization's mission and values as transformation from a culture of volume to value.

Main Theme 2: Customer and Market Focus

According to the Malcolm Baldrige model, an organization's focus on the customer and market further satisfied the expectations of the customer. This category examined how the leaders proactively engaged the voice of their customers and used customer feedback to identify opportunities for improvement. Questions 8-12 examined how the leaders engage patients and use their feedback to increase the value of care delivered. Question eight was designed to understand how leaders improved the value of care for their patients while Questions nine and 11 probed how leaders responded to their customers' expectations without becoming overwhelmed. Questions 10 and 12 questioned how much of customers' expectations affected quality improvement initiatives and if it was possible to focus both on the patient and the financial bottom line. Coding and analysis within the customer focus category identified participants believed methods to improve value for patients should focus on patient satisfaction, patient engagement, and patient education.

Patient Satisfaction.

Participants agreed a focus on methods to satisfy patients increased both the value of care provided and the strength of the company. Participants believed a commitment to patient satisfaction will promote activities and habits rooted in value because of a change in attitudes. These activities, according to participants, continued to produce the greatest outcomes in relation to the resources spent as employees would be focused on the level of care delivered and organizational use of resources to deliver the care. These activities consisted of reducing fragmentation of care through efficient use of resources such as technology and engaging employees to learn best practices or to make appropriate decisions in the best interest of the patient. One participant provided an example that sometimes employees had attitudes that stressed quality and patient satisfaction at all costs. This participant highlighted that leaders needed to have crucial conversations with employees to deliver the message that 'cost does not equal quality.'

One participant believed patients valued cost more than quality because patients wanted high quality of care; more importantly, patients wanted to be able to afford quality health care. Participants commented patient education is of key importance to satisfying a patient's expectations. Participants said patients benefited from clinical improvement measures that organizations implemented. One participant believed leaders should not be concerned with patient satisfaction as an indicator of the value of services provided. Instead, this participant voiced that organizational leaders should be attentive to improving clinical process measures whose outcomes would have more value to patients than satisfying the patients. Another participant noted, although leaders should engage in activities that satisfy the patient, leaders should not feel pressured to respond to all patients' demands. The key element is to ensure patients were aware the organization valued the patient's input.

Patient Engagement.

In addition to satisfying patients with improved clinical outcomes at reduced costs, participants viewed patient engagement as a source of data that provides insight to patient's expectations. Twenty out of 21 participants shared the importance of patient engagement and the use of their feedback to improve clinical outcomes and optimizing organizational processes to ensure outcomes are satisfactory to patients. No one admitted to underperformance in any areas except one participant who stated that organizations did not perform well in many areas and would benefit from patient engagement for two reasons: to highlight areas that needed improving and to demonstrate the commitment to increasing the quality of care. One participant emphasized active engagement allowed patients to participate more in their own health care processes, which increased provider's efficiency. Patient engagement was reflected in the responses and was considered the best source of information and needed to be taken seriously.

Patient Education.

One participant stressed, as part of a focus on the patients, organizational leaders not only need to listen to a patient's feedback, or give them an opportunity to participate in their care, but patients also need to be educated. The participant commented, not achieving a clinical quality outcome should not be blamed on a non-compliant patient or a defect in the process of care. Instead, patient education should be considered. According to the participant, through patient education, patients were knowledgeable on best practices. That knowledge that contributed to an increased quality of life as patients were more aware of their own lifestyle decisions. Education promoted healthier people and amplified the positive outcomes of clinical care.

Secondary data analysis indicated organizations described quality in a similar manner to participants, that was, safe and excellent. Content analysis revealed that organizations were focused on providing high-quality, health-care based on CMS's organizational requirements and based on the organization's reputation through transparency of the organization's actions.

Main Theme 3: Workforce Focus

According to the Malcolm Baldrige model, the Workforce Focus category examined how leaders engaged and developed employees to create an environment of high performance and accomplish organization's goals. For this study, Questions 13-17 examined how the leaders communicated and promoted the vision of value-based care to its workforce. This category also reflected how leadership motivated and transformed the environment to one based on value that was capable of meeting new health-care goals. Interview Questions 13-17 were designed to understand the frequency of training needed to promote value-based culture (Question 13), how leaders develop employees to increase their efficiency (Question 14), understand resource allocation to develop the workforce (Question 15), how change is introduced without causing frustration (Question 14), and how leaders should incentivize employees to change their attitudes from volume-based culture to one of value (Question 17).

After coding and analysis against the workforce focus category, it was evident the leaders promoted the vision through training and education that also transformed attitudes and work habits in the work environment. In addition to training and education, leaders also incentivized their employees to change behaviors.

Employee Efficiency.

Employee efficiency, according to participants, leads to sustained excellence. Six out of 21 participants focused on the need for training in value-based practices, while an additional five participants noted both training and education were means to increasing efficiency. Ten out of 21 participants discussed the importance of hiring personnel with appropriate skills and shared values, observation and feedback, and sharing of information as ways to increase efficiency. Based on responses, these elements made employees more aware of their actions and unnecessary costs and/or patient events occur so employees could make better decisions in the future.

Resource Allocation.

Another element of creating value for the organization was resource allocation to develop and transform the workforce. Although two participants noted it was unwise for leaders to place any constraints on resources used to train and develop employees, 19 out of 21 participants believed the number of resources invested in the workforce should be in proportion to the amount of value-based initiatives applied. Two participants specifically seemed more conservative and offered that leaders should find creative ways to develop the workforce as opposed to excessive usage of resources. An example of one creative opportunity was conducting meetings during the lunch hour so patient care was not delayed. Another example was hiring the most qualified, well-suited, and skilled personnel, therefore reducing the number of resources invested in the category of workforce training.

Prevention of Frustration.

Employee frustration was not explicitly addressed in the Malcolm Baldrige model, but its lack thereof may reduce the expectations of value-based strategies implemented. It was assumed, given the amount of legislative changes occurring in health care, employees may become frustrated and easily overwhelmed. Legal changes were another important area to for leaders to share their experience in curbing frustration. Participants' responses to, "How best is it to introduce (legal, policy, procedural) change without causing frustration from staff?" (Question 16) presented the role leaders had in transformation of the culture to one that was value-based and promotion of behaviors that could result in quality outcomes. Participants shared that it may not be inevitable, but it was apparent measures were undertaken to ease the frustration in response the change to value-based principles. One participant mentioned it was easy for leaders to overwhelm and frustrate employees because leaders get 'caught in the swirl' as they attempt to focus on too many initiatives simultaneously. As a means of preventing frustration, leaders could offer the benefit of retreats where senior leaders ensured the leaders' actions were focused and aligned to the organization's goals. Leaders could also share a consistent message with staff. Other measures offered by participants included leaders' communication of organization's goals and expectations, providing reasons for what was being done, and employee engagement.

Training.

Despite the need for training to increase the value of care delivered to patients, participants varied considerably in their responses for frequency of training. Eighteen out of 21 responses varied from the needs being daily, as needed, once a year, several times a year as new initiatives were implemented, quarterly, and/or continual until the organization was comfortable with the results. One participant offered a differing opinion and stated the focus should not be on the frequency of training stating, but ensuring employees understood the basic principles of value-based care; and to dismiss employees if they could not comprehend or act on such principles. Another participant did not share a specific time frame and offered the opinion that frequency of training is dependent on the culture of the organization. One participant shared that some people with an intrinsic desire to help others sought jobs in health care. Therefore, such people already have the desire to perform better, so did not require as much training.

Incentivizing Behavior.

Three participants' responses reflected they believed employees had an innate desire to seek continuous improvement. These participants reflected on the reasons they personally entered a health-care profession and shared their reasons. Those personal reasons included a desire to help someone, to work effectively, and to contribute to society. These participants believed if employees were reminded of the reasons they chose health care as their profession, they would naturally perform better. One participant believed if leaders were to hire individuals who shared similar values to those of the organization, then leaders would not have to concentrate on incentivizing behavior. Another five out of 21 participants believed the culture affected behavior more than incentives. Only six out of 21 responses considered employees' need for immediate gratification, which included the use of company-sponsored food, gain-sharing, awards, praise, and words of appreciation. One participant cautioned it was important to incentivize behaviors only when outcomes were met; another stated value-based behavior should be an expectation as part of a daily routine and not something to be incentivized. The other four participants discussed involving the workforce in decision-making and contributing to the solution so the employees are incentivized to achieve the desired outcomes.

Main Theme 4: Strategic Planning

The Malcolm Baldrige criteria examined the development of action plans to achieve organizational goals, how plans are modified should circumstances change, and the resources dedicated to implement such plans. It is how organizations prepared for continued sustenance. This preparation was accomplished through establishment of short and long-term goals. Question 18-22 related to sustained performance excellence in value-based health care in areas of cost-effectiveness, efficiency, and sustainability (Questions 18, 19, & 20). This category also examined how leaders allocated resources to support implementation strategies that reflected elements of cost-effectiveness, efficiency, and sustainability (Questions 21 & 22).

A common finding was participants believed sustainability meant a balance between providing high quality care that satisfied the customer, as well as having revenues that exceeded expenses. A noteworthy observation was the overwhelming number of responses to the number of cost-effective strategies as a means of sustainability. Leaders expressed these strategies could increase the value of care provided and increase the probability of earning the maximum reimbursement for services provided. Participant suggestions for cost-effective strategies were noted as follows:

- *Integration of care*: doctors, the health plan, and the facilities (work environment) all worked together towards a common goal versus trying to partner with different people in different organizations.
- *Knowledge and discussion of costs*: This

increased awareness was for problematic areas in which to increase efficiency.

- *Cost Standardization:* reduced variance in cost of procedures and medical supplies that would, in turn, decrease unnecessary expenditure.
- *Evaluation of specific areas of clinical care:* a focus on specific areas shed light on clinical areas to improve
- *Communication:* increased discussion that resulted in creative cost-effective strategies.
- *Process Improvement Strategies:* helped evaluate consistency in quality and identified areas defective or opportunities for further improvement. A focus on specific processes increased effectiveness at improving deficient areas and maximized use of resource(s). Strategies such as Lean and Six Sigma could be used to examine all processes in depth that provided data on each step and high-expenditure areas where costs could be reduced.
- *Decrease clinical variation:* standardization in health care processes
- *Use of shared decision-making process:* Providers and patients can evaluate treatment plans before consenting to treatment that could reduce waste.
- *Leadership Visibility and Involvement:* ability to continuously spread the vision, sharing of information, and ability to provide feedback to employees as the staff worked

- *Culture of Continuous Improvement*: There was always room for improvement.
- *Use of a Quality Dashboard*: use of a dashboard to evaluate and assess quality and outcome indicators selected based on specific areas of quality focus
- *Engagement of Employees*: involve those who carry out the clinical work in decision-making processes
- *Patient and Patient Caregiver Education*: Success of process measures was dependent on patients' involvement and understanding of their treatment plan. Education helped patients manage their home health care that prevented unnecessary visits to and from multiple health-care providers.
- *Operations Strategies*: effective use of resources, leverage technology to reduce costs, automate as much as possible, evaluate areas for process redesign, effective use of data
- *Inventory Management:* reduce costs through better management of supplies stored onsite
- *Labor Management*: Increased productivity as employees practice to the extent of their duties/qualifications (licensing); individuals could focus on their job as opposed to others filling the work or task (void) at a higher expense.
- *Creativity in Care Delivery*: Seek less expensive alternatives versus a hospital stay, e.g., at home care, online through virtual care, in an ambulatory setting, prevention of admission and readmission, and/or improving office visit processes.

- *Use of Cost Accounting System*: This method provided working data on previous and current costs that organizations could keep revisiting to find further ways of increasing cost-efficiency.
- *Reallocation of Labor*: Employees can be placed in different departments or function in a different capacity to avoid lay-offs because of budget constraints.
- *Use of Specific Cost Measurement Strategies*: examples include a feedback process, patient management strategy. Use of these specific cost measurements could narrow highlighted areas of improvement and reduce resources and expenditure.
- *Benchmark:* provided the ability to see what other organizations are doing for efficiency
- *Use of A3 Thinking:* allowed leaders to focus on one area and costs associated with it.
- *Stakeholder Education*: Maximized resources' use through education of the provider and the patient on process improvement.
- *Accountability:* responsible to reduce costs, even if processes exceeded standards

One participant said there was no need to have a specific strategy to increase efficiency; leaders needed to review processes and stop any service of processes that did not provide any value to patients.

Strategy Resource Allocation.

Answers to additional probing as to how to prevent becoming overambitious in developing strategies were collected in Question 21. All participants recognized resource allocation was very important in strategic planning. Four out of 21 participants expressed prevention of over-ambition in planning and allocating resources was a challenge. The rest of participants offered multiple methods to curb over-ambition. These included, prioritization of tasks, standardizing work processes, use of a planning dashboard, use of benchmarking, and keeping mission-focused, while looking for simple solutions to maximize resources. Participants voiced the importance of knowing what the organizational costs are and continuously seeking ways to improve, especially through leveraging the use of technology to streamline and automate processes. One significant example of a cost-efficient strategy was described as having employees *practice on top of their license* (defined as a labor resource maximized for a standard workflow as transfer of care is shifted between providers).

Main Theme 5: Operation Focus

The Operation Focus category of the Malcolm Baldrige criteria referred to the approach that health-care leaders used to identify core competencies to achieve efficient and effective management of operations. Interview Questions 23-25 related to processes used to improve the organization's work system, meaning, how leaders ensured performance excellence and reflection of value in its services. Questions were: "What are the processes used to shift the focus to value in care as opposed to increasing volume" (Question 23), "What are some destructive effects of value-based health care on operations," and (Question 24), "What do you consider to be operation efficiency" (Question 25).

Optimizing Operations to Value.

Commonly, reports focused on business process improvement and outcomes for patients. Participants stated the need for evaluation of outcomes, improvement of patient experience, and efficient use of resources as the processes used to shift the focus to value in care. An emphasis on optimizing care and operational processes as well as improving the value for patients were repeated themes in participant's responses. Based on their responses, participants had a sharp focus on ensuring clinical outcomes were of high quality and met patient's expectations. Another method to optimize operations was to focus on increasing efficiency. All participants viewed efficiency as the absence of waste. One participant added efficiency also meant how quickly patients had significant improvement of their quality of life.

Preparation for Success.

Responses to the question of the destructive effects of value-based care (Question 24), participants noted there was uncertainty adopting a pay-for-performance culture. Participants offered ideas for opportunity to avoid experiencing these destructive effects. These ideas included the right combination of subject matter expertise to ensure the program was implemented appropriately, improvement of processes with the patient in mind, and education of key stakeholders so everyone shared the same vision.

Main Theme 6: Measurement, Analysis, and Knowledge

This category of the Malcolm Baldrige Criteria examined how leaders integrated additional information to review and improved organizational performance and outcomes. The category also examined how leaders used resources to facilitate decision-making and maintenance of a competitive position with other health-care organizations.

Specifically, for value-based health care, Interview Questions 26-28 examined how leaders integrate data improved organizational performance and used resources to facilitate value-focused decision-making and maintenance of a competitive position. The questions in this category were, "How important is integrating data to improving efficiency"

(Question 26), "What is the best way to use performance findings to change or improve work processes for better efficiency" (Question, 27), and "How do you devote resources to this venture" (Question 28). Coding and analysis within this category identified the need to integrate data and description of ways to allocate resources efficiently.

Data Integration.

The general agreement to data integration was a very important task organizations should be part of in an organization's strategic plan. Participants agreed there was not one perfect approach, but the key is to improve with resources available and to be specific as to what goals organizations were trying to achieve. Participants shared similar responses – it was important to evaluate process and outcomes to provide feedback if improvement had occurred. The most popular response of data integration was benchmarking. Based on participants' responses, it was clear that plans on whether to, or how to, benchmark seemed dependent on the organization's work-place culture. Three participants warned that leaders should be conscious of its suitability and applicability and how the data pertained to their organizational environment. One participant voiced that organizations should not benchmark, because it could prevent organizations from extending their financial capabilities beyond expected organizational standards. Another participant shared the idea that leaders should look at non-health care industries and evaluate areas approach to excellence, especially in high-risk areas.

Measurement Resource Allocation.

Participants stressed using resources responsibly and efficiently in response to how resources were devoted to finding and comparing data (Question 28). Of the participants, 15 out of 21 noted the number of resources devoted to measurement and analysis was dependent on availability of resources. Although five out of 21 participants acknowledged there was difficulty in allocating resources appropriately, at least one participant said, to achieve certain quality and costs outcomes, leaders should prioritize their organizations' goals and work with resources available. One participant believed a lack of resources did not limit an organization's ability to increase their capabilities. The participant advised organizations form collaborations as a method to share resources.

Main Theme 7: Results

This category examined how an organization performed in the rest of the Malcolm Baldrige categories – in areas of process efficiency, preparedness, and operational effectiveness that impacted the outcomes for the customers. Performance in these areas was especially important to financial sustainability and accomplishment of strategic goals as a participant of Medicare's value-based health care program. Questions 29-33 examined the performance of the organization that lead to results such as financial sustainability and accomplishment of strategic goals. The questions were, "What key data is necessary to set performance targets"(Question 29), "How often should performance results be reviewed"(Question 30), "How should success in Medicare's value-based health care be measured" (Question 31), " How are unintended consequences avoided" (Question 32), and "Is there any area that you think is important to address as organizations try to find the balance between achieving high quality while lowering costs and remaining financially viable" (Question 33).

Cultural Influence.

Four participants believed the time frame was dependent on the organization's objectives, what was measured, and the culture of the organization.

Seventeen out of 21 provided responses such as "patient satisfaction," "accounts receivable," "readmission rates," "change in health status," and "aggregate spending," which were reflective of a focus on the patient or the organization. One participant recognized the need to maintain a balance of focus for the patient and organization when setting performance targets, stating some performance targets like length of stay was of no value to the patient, but important to the bottom line. Responses to the frequency in which performance results should be reviewed varied from daily, monthly, quarterly, every six months, and yearly. Participants agreed that performance should be reviewed in three basic elements; quality, service, and costs. The key lesson implied from participants was that measurement of results occurred at some point that provides indication of performance and operational effectiveness. Leaders may have to decide if they could have intervened earlier to produce more desirable patient satisfaction results.

Success.

Based on responses to "How should success in Medicare's value-based health care be measured?" (Question 31), it was apparent participants shared a strong commitment to the achievement of the organization's cost-reduction and patient care goals. This commitment reflected an acceptance to hospital leadership change and allowed value-based behaviors to permeate the health-care industry. Achievement of metrics and satisfactory outcomes, both clinically and financially, summarized participant's view of success in value-based care. Use of metrics not only helped in evaluating whether outcomes were met, but also provided a set of baseline data that organizations could use to continue to improve. In comparing the primary data answers from participants and the secondary data sources, only one participant identified the use of revenue as a measure of success.

Plan for Success

Question 32 elicited responses of undesirable consequences and received responses of mixed feelings. Though leader participants mentioned several potential destructive effects, a few immediately followed responses with 'comfort words' such as, "… you have to bounce back," and "… just be prepared," although others seemed more critical of the current design of Medicare's value-based health care program. Participants were critical the societal culture was not willing to change from one of volume to value since the health-care system was motivated by profit, patients were misinformed, and inappropriate decisions made by clinicians. No participants specifically described an experience of an unintended consequence. It was evident these answers were full of emotion and seemed more theoretical in nature as participants tried to weigh the advantages and disadvantages of the value-based program. One participant advised implementation of risk mitigation plans to avoid reduce those risks and unintended consequences.

Considerations of Value-Based Health Care.

The intent of Question 33 was to shed light on potential to consider as health-care organizations transform to a value-based culture. About 90% of respondents hesitated before responding, though the other 10% already had ideas of potential defects in the program. Issues participants commented on, but was not addressed by the researcher, were as follows:

- A reluctance by leaders to share information and have conversations about costs with key stakeholders out of fear of having to point fingers (who made the mistake?), rather than learning lessons from an unfortunate event.
- Earning less revenue due to recession; patients were unemployed therefore unable to pay their health-benefit co-pays. This inability to pay plus the added burden of having payments withheld from Medicare created anxiety.
- Continuance of non-beneficial activities to patients despite the national initiative to increase the value

of care for patients.

- The uncertainty of whether patient satisfaction could be measured. The issue arose when patients demanded services not necessarily in their best interest.
- Lack of personal (patient) accountability. Organizations could develop and implement stellar strategies rooted in value; however, if patients are not held accountable for their lifestyle choices or health care decisions, why should the organization be penalized for not meeting clinical outcomes? One participant equated how car insurance is calculated in terms of many people can control the things that gave a negative health outcome and how do policy makers strongly discourage people (patients) from choosing the lifestyle that leads to poorer health outcomes.
- Pay-for-performance/value was not the appropriate answer for sustained improvement in health care. Managed care was offered as a more appropriate model.
- Length of time it took for organizations to be reimbursed; long wait time put a greater strain on the health-care organization's finances.
- Motivation of putting patients first is missing; organizations need to focus more on sustaining themselves; patients cannot be the focus.
- Many unknowns in the program may take too long to be addressed and result in unnecessary waste of resources.

Presentation of Secondary Data

The analysis presented in this chapter was also based on using content analysis with public published documents from five random healthcare organizations. These documents were reviewed for ways organizations sought ways to improve the delivery of care and their processes to facilitate a more efficient industry with greater health care outcomes for their patients using the same categories of the Malcolm Baldrige Criteria.

Leadership

No specific secondary data were found regarding the methods to share the vision of value-based health care and get a 'buy-in' without overwhelming the staff. Organizational documents reviewed implied organizations shared a common vision of improving care and lowering costs, but were not specific on the actions of leaders. One organization mentioned it used the Malcolm Baldrige tool as a guideline for improvement in organizations, so it was concluded data supported the participant's views of leadership roles.

Customer Focus

Responses to the interview questions that triangulated with content analysis of the organizational documents strongly suggested health-care organizations needed to focus primarily on the patient. Although documents revealed several strategies of ways the organization is improving to care for patients, there was no specific mention of a benefit to the organization. Organizations portrayed their efforts for improvement were in the interest of making people healthier. All documents reflected similar perceptions of participant's responses to quality. Safety, meeting quality measures, and excellent outcomes were words used to describe the quality of care provided within secondary data. One organization added a high-quality organization is defined as the best place to heal and could be equated to satisfactory outcomes participants described. Participants and secondary data identified quality in terms of the health care provided to patients; however, it was evident that organizations also highlight quality in terms of their business reputation and institution's accreditation status. This was derived from data from three out of five organizations that emphasized the experience of the physicians, services provided, and awards received as indicators of quality. Participants did not discuss awards or reputation (referencing quality).

The body of secondary data corroborated the participants' responses on engaging patients to enlist their feedback to improve organizational processes. Four out of the five organizations provided additional insights on how they engage patients through surveys and how much they relied on that information to assess their services. They shared a commitment to improve care for patients through use of clinical guidelines and provision of satisfactory experiences. Two out of the five organizational documents highlighted efforts to reduce costs for the patients as a means of improving value to them. All the health-care organizations, except one, shared similar views; increasing value is a way of delivering satisfactory outcomes. The outlier organization associated value with outcomes of care experienced by the patients.

It was also evident health-care organizations valued feedback from patients – similar to participants' responses. Organizations shared they use patient information to guide initiatives and improvements. Three out of the five organizations also referenced initiatives to promote good health and quality of life as an indicator of the health care institution's commitment to improve lives within the community. This was achieved through free health seminars or partnering with organizations such as the YMCA, offering free vaccinations, and/or involvement with community events that highlighted healthy choice decision-making.

Workforce Focus

There was no explicit data on how organizations trained and developed their workforce, or incentivized behaviors. It was observed in all five organizations there was a strong attempt to maintain high levels of employee satisfaction indicated from statements such as "best place to work," "best environment," and "work/life balance." Three out of the four organizations encouraged continuing education by offering tuition reimbursements or scholarships. One organization had a dedicated online university that offered learning activities to further enhance the clinical employees' abilities in general areas.

Measurement, Analysis, and Knowledge

Participants believed leaders should use outside data to compare their practices in specific areas compared to the community, through benchmarking. It was evident, from the body of secondary data, the health-care organizations valued comparing themselves to competitors to ensure a focus on best practices. The observed organizations believed their practices in clinical areas set the standard for other health-care competitors to emulate. Organizations such as LeapFrog and Hospital Compare were cited as comparative data sources. Of note, the secondary data triangulated participants' emphasis on the importance of benchmarking. Referencing participants' advice, the theme was to be cautious of benchmarking and its applicability. Documents did not reflect this theme of caution.

Operation Focus

The secondary data was not specific to the organization's approach to achieve effective and efficient operations. The secondary data interpreted that organizations referred to their own mission, vision, and values as their operation focus as most documents made references to these statements. Values reflected a commitment to strive for high levels of operational, financial performance and improving services for patients. Statistical highlights supported statements, especially in the finance area. These same mission and values drove this research study's participants; therefore, the secondary data triangulated to their responses.

Strategy Planning

Documents reviewed did not triangulate the specific strategies to sustaining cost-efficiency in the organizations compared to what participants revealed. The organization's strategic plans focused on continuous improvement to provide the best care for the patients. Documents reflected plans for the organization's growth, including the addition of services or forming collaborations with other organizations to meet the health needs of the community.

Results

Based on the focus of multiple awards and accolades, organizations seem to have met their clinical outcomes. There was no indication that organizations lacked in clinical quality performance. Two out of the five organizations acknowledged changes in the health-care industry and perseverance to strive to deliver the best for the health-care organization's patients. Three out of the five organizations had committed to increasing efficiency interpreted as reducing costs for both patient and the organization.

Chapter Summary

This chapter presented data gathered from participant's responses to the interview questions structured to answer the main research question. The research question addressed the best business strategies health-care leaders used to increase the value of care for success by health-care organizations in Medicare's value-based health care program.

Using the Malcolm Baldrige criteria as a quality improvement tool, the results were summarized in Figure 3. Data analysis of the participants' responses indicated some leaders did not recognize the term value-based health care, but all research-study participants revealed they had worked with various strategies to accomplish goals of improving health care at lower costs for the benefit of the patient and/or the organization. The sub-question of the main research question addressed how leaders balanced between increasing the value of care, lowering costs, and sustained organizational financial growth. Analysis of the data revealed an integration of strategies influenced by the organizations' workplace culture, and resources that fostered alignment with the health-care organization's clinical and business goals. Participants believed the leader's role was critical to guiding employees to deliver the kind of care envisioned and ultimately leading the organization to success. The researcher noticed more similarities than differences between the secondary data reviewed and data obtained from participants' responses to the interview questions. Of the categories, secondary data strongly supported participants' responses in the customer focus category.

CORE VALUE-BASED STRATEGIC OBJECTIVES

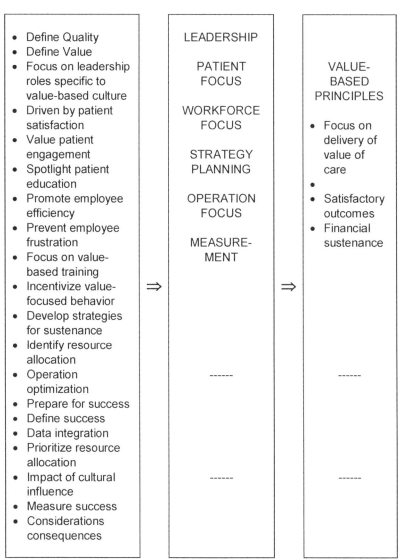

- Define Quality
- Define Value
- Focus on leadership roles specific to value-based culture
- Driven by patient satisfaction
- Value patient engagement
- Spotlight patient education
- Promote employee efficiency
- Prevent employee frustration
- Focus on value-based training
- Incentivize value-focused behavior
- Develop strategies for sustenance
- Identify resource allocation
- Operation optimization
- Prepare for success
- Define success
- Data integration
- Prioritize resource allocation
- Impact of cultural influence
- Measure success
- Considerations consequences

LEADERSHIP

PATIENT FOCUS

WORKFORCE FOCUS

STRATEGY PLANNING

OPERATION FOCUS

MEASURE-MENT

$\Rightarrow$

VALUE-BASED PRINCIPLES

- Focus on delivery of value of care
-
- Satisfactory outcomes
- Financial sustenance

$\Rightarrow$

Figure 3 - Value-based strategies using Baldrige Criteria

Further analysis was presented in Chapter 5 with a discussion of the results and proposes a framework adapted from the Baldrige Criteria for Performance Excellence in the conclusions. A discussion of the limitations and implications of the study and recommendations for further research concluded Chapter 5.

Chapter 5

Discussion, Implications, Recommendations

The purpose of this qualitative study was to explore the best strategies leadership personnel deemed necessary for health-care organizations to operate efficiently to deliver high quality services rooted in value. This research could be of significance for the health-care organizations looking for a fresh approach to use resources appropriately to reduce waste, increase value of services, deliver the quality of health care the system as intended, and be able to maintain their financial status. The results of this study support the need for evidence-based business strategies that facilitates success in participating organizations of Medicare's value-based program and a redefinition of financial sustainability in health care that emphasizes value.

This chapter presents a review and conclusion obtained from the research study's findings and recommendations for health-care leaders to understand the business strategies that contribute to increasing the value of clinical outcomes. The chapter is organized according to (a) Evaluation of Methodological Approach, (b) Contextual Background of the Study, (c) Discussion of Results, (d) Implications, and (e) Recommendations for Future Research.

Evaluation of Methodological Approach

A qualitative case study was deemed appropriate for this research because the purpose of the study was exploratory in nature and required the ability to be fluid. Such a methodology permits the researcher to gain detailed information about value-based health care by using interviews and publicly available, published documents on the health-care organizations' quality improvement. A qualitative study allows the researcher to assimilate and understand the numerous factors that underlie value-based health care. This methodology also allows the researcher to generate an in-depth description of business strategies organizations use to support value-based health care and maintain organizational financial viability from participants' perspectives.

An exploratory case study was appropriate as it allows the researcher to explore the lack of business strategies specific to value-based health and use participants' responses and text within secondary data as the units of analysis. The case study approach facilitated thematic analysis that provides the researcher an opportunity to deliver a holistic and in-depth understanding of the multiple perspectives obtained on value-based health care.

Contextual Background

To understand and analyze the data findings, the previous chapters are summarized in the following section to develop a contextual background of the study. Chapter one provided a detailed introduction of the issues of waste, and unnecessary costs in health care that cause concern for sustainability of the health-care system. A discussion of Medicare's current focus efficiency and value of care for patients through implementation of a reimbursement program based on value and performance outcomes ensued. Chapter one contained a discussion of a need for further refinement of Medicare's value-based program. The problem identified in the current program is the program provides an incomplete model for holistic improvement. The model only provides measures of quality clinical outcomes and leaves leaders within health-care organizations to blindly determine the best business strategies to promote success in the Medicare's value-based program. This chapter offers further discussion for the significance of this research study is that a lack of knowledge of a health-care organization's business practices that encourages success is an impediment to sustenance of financial improvement in the health-care industry. Presented in Chapter 1 were the researcher's assumptions, limitations, and definition of terms. The chapter concluded with an introduction of the use of the Malcolm Baldrige Criteria for Performance Excellence whose purpose is to guide organizational performance, as a quality improvement tool for answering the research study's questions.

A review of the literature in Chapter 2 revealed the reasons for issues of waste and inefficiency in health care. An overview of quality improvement strategies used to address these issues over the decades was provided. Past and current strategies highlighted specific areas of focus such as the patient, processes, outcomes, and quality of product or services as individual elements to improvement. Despite the advantages of several models of quality improvement, continued efforts to improve did not deliver sustained improvement because previous goals did not emphasize value as the underlying driver for health improvement. There was no stimulus for meaningful change; health-care organizations were paid regardless of the quality of their health-care services. The industry's attitudes of focusing on earning revenue affected not only patients, but also payers of health-care services. As a result, one of the largest payers of health-care services, Medicare, took on pecuniary measures of motivation to encourage health-care reform. The goal of this federal-level measure was to increase the value of health care provided to patients and to improve the patient's clinical quality in outcomes per dollars spent. The underlying principles of this effort are reliant on efficiency, cost containment, and increased quality of life in patients. Medicare's value-based program only addressed the clinical aspects – and not the entire health-care system. Considerable empirical evidence exists to suggest that strategies geared towards non-clinical structural and process activities lead to improved business performance (Sila, 2007; Yaacob, 2010). This lack of knowledge can hinder a health-care organization's efforts towards clinical quality improvement, as well as increase the probability of losing Medicare reimbursements, hence, the purpose for this research.

The study used the Malcolm Baldrige Criteria for Performance Excellence as the conceptual framework for this exploratory case study. The literature reviewed by this study's researcher illustrated the Malcolm Baldrige Criteria for Performance Excellence model promotes the principles of TQM, leads to positive outcomes in performance and quality, and serves as a catalyst to reshape attitudes and behavior toward quality improvement. The researcher discussed the use of the Malcolm Baldrige Model for Performance Excellence as a tool to put into practice the elements of TQM in a value-based health environment. The researcher expected that participants' responses would identify strategies specific to value-based health care using the Malcolm Baldrige criteria as a guideline. Through a summary of studies, the literature review highlighted that the use of the Malcolm Baldrige model allowed integration of a wide range of strategies beyond those that focus solely on clinical health-care quality outcomes and presented successful outcomes to the organization with its use.

Presented in chapter 3 were an overview of the exploratory qualitative case study methodology chosen for this research and a detailed review of the research design. Methods taken to collect data included conducting a field test to ensure the interview questions elicited appropriate answers to the research questions. A summary of the researcher's experience was provided. A discussion of the Malcolm Baldrige Criteria for Performance Excellence was the model against which to compare the instrument followed. An overview of secondary data sources used to assist in triangulation and corroboration of themes from the primary data source was added. Issues of validity and reliability of the study, to include the researcher's experience, and methods taken to ensure protection of participants concluded the chapter.

In Chapter 4, a description of the sample was provided, which included 21 participants of leaders and included executive, middle, and frontline managers in a variety of leadership roles and years in quality improvement experience. The chapter included an explanation of the data collection process, followed by a presentation of participants' responses to the semi-structured interview questions. In this chapter, the interview data were also triangulated with secondary data gathered from publically available documents from the healthcare industry such as financial reports, organizational executive summaries, strategic development documents, and quality reports. The intent of Chapter

5 is to discuss the findings in response to the research questions, implications, conclusions, and provide recommendations for future research.

Discussion of Results

Chapter 4 presented the findings of the primary data and triangulated these findings with secondary data. Analysis of participants' responses and secondary data revealed common sub-themes within each category of the Baldrige model. The categories of the Baldrige model were used as predefined themes. The following is an evaluation of these data identified from responses to the 33 interview questions.

Research Question 1

The purpose of the main research question is to understand the business strategies health-care leaders use to increase the value of care for patients for success in Medicare's value-based health care program. Success was viewed as receiving maximum reimbursement from Medicare for service(s) provided. A review of respondents' data revealed this research study's participants focus on multiple strategies that improve the value of care delivered, increased efficiency and accountability of practices and services, and sustain quality improvement in health care. This finding was in alignment with previous research that suggests strategies geared toward non-clinical structural and process activities also lead to improved business performance, as indicated by increased efficiency and effectiveness of services and products, which ultimately results in improved financial performance (Sila, 2007; Yaacob, 2010).

Discussion of Leadership Findings

Leadership category in the Malcolm Baldrige model addressed how leaders manage and guide their system to performance excellence and sustainability in value-based health care. It included how leaders communicate and promote the vision of value and quality to the organization's stakeholders. This category also reflected how leaders transform the environment to one that is capable of meeting new health care goals by changing the culture from a volume-based to a value-based business model and motivation of the workforce.

Based on participants' tone of voice, body language (for in-person interviews) and length of answers; participants seemed passionate about the subject and eager to answer the questions. A possible explanation for such eagerness could be the relative newness of the value-based concept and the urgency to develop practices rooted in value, as organizations are at risk for losing Medicare revenue should the healthcare-organization fail at achieving clinical outcomes.

A significant theme that strongly supports the Malcolm Baldrige model and previous research from Tralib and Rahman (2010) is the commitment of health-care organization leaders to promote quality output and sustained excellence. Research participants noted leaders have the responsibility to ensure care is delivered in a satisfactory manner to the patients, as well as efficiently to ensure financial sustainability of the health-care organization. These participant's views indicated leaders within the organization play a critical role in implementing business strategies supportive of value-based care and promotion of service excellence in the quality of care delivered.

Based on participants' responses, it is through communication of the vision, expectations, goals, and the status of goal achievement that health-care organization leaders influence the quality of work and clinical outcomes. Consequently, employees are more aware of methods to increase the value of care for patients and are more attentive to increasing efficiency. Therefore, optimal outcomes are produced with limited variance. From participants' responses, the researcher sensed health-care organization leaders were putting forth their best efforts to ensure operations were cost-efficient, especially as health-care organizations are no longer paid for by Medicare for the volume of services. Health-care organization leaders seemed committed to increasing the value of service provided to patients. Content analysis of the secondary data – that is the documents reviewed – implied health-care leaders within the organizations are responsible and committed to transforming the health-care industry to sustained improvement through refining (business) care processes and becoming more patient-centric. These results lend support to the relationship between communication and organizational performance as promoted by the Malcolm Baldrige model, as well as support the notion health-care organization leaders are the drivers that guide the sustained pursuit of quality and performance objectives (NIST, 2013) within the industry.

Discussion of Customer Focus Findings

The Customer and Market Focus category in the Malcolm Baldrige model examined how health-care organization leaders proactively engaged the customers' feedback and use patient feedback to identify areas to increase the value of care provided. The category also examined how leaders adapt operations to ensure the health-care products and services satisfy and meet customer expectations. From the literature review, quality improvement strategies emphasized satisfying the customer (Suarez, 1992). This focus on satisfying the customer continues to be the highlight in current quality improvement models. Tralib and Rahman (2010) postulated it is essential for leaders within organizations to understand customers' needs through feedback; they purported it is the essence of organizational success. This research study's results support the previous findings of the importance of the customer (patient) as a means of organizational excellence. It was apparent the patient is the driving force of the organization. Responses indicated participants believed satisfying customers' expectations is a combination of giving the customer a voice, in addition to bearing the ethical responsibility to doing what is right. The research study's participants' responses implied the reasons for engaging patients to participate actively in discussions, regarding their care and satisfaction, are more effective than assuming the quality level of health care needed.

An interesting concept presented in a review of the data was of educating patients about their processes of care, not only to make better life choices to improve their quality of life, but also to facilitate the success of organization's clinical improvement initiatives. Stone et al. (2010) discussed findings of the impact of predisposing patient factors to quality outcomes, but did not suggest education as a means of sustaining quality and satisfaction outcomes. Participants voiced concern patients do not always benefit from measures implemented, because of the decisions the patients make regarding their own health. Patient satisfaction scores and outcomes in specific areas of clinical care are part of the Medicare reimbursement calculation. Patient education could be a very effective approach to improving outcomes and prevent health-care organizations from being penalized because of a patient's irresponsibility or lack of compliance from ignorance about their health conditions or care of the same. If health-care organizations implemented a quality care process and outcome measures, these outcomes may not be valid without proper patient education.

Research-study participants were also in agreement the best interest of patients is to incentivize the patients to live a healthier lifestyle. Research-study participants recognized the impact such that patients will not need the health-care organization's services. An interesting suggestion was that – as part of industry improvement – organizational leaders will possess the responsibility to prevent hospital admissions by making patients healthier. Consequently, participants noted health-care, organizational leaders will need to find other ways of sustaining the longevity of the organization, such as providing home-health or virtual care. Secondary data reflected a movement to new methods of making patients healthier by becoming more involved in their home health care via the use of Internet technology.

Discussion of Workforce Focus Findings

The Workforce Focus category in the Malcolm Baldrige model examined how leaders communicate and promote the vision of value to health-care employees. The workforce category probed the strategies that health-care leaders employ to transform the workplace environment to one capable of meeting new business and clinical goals through changing the culture and motivating the workforce. Research showed, to build quality and organizational excellence, a focus should be on the employees within the organization (Dahlgaard et al., 2011; Jayamaha et al., 2008; Yaacob, 2010). Within this category, research-study participants supported the need to focus on the workforce and implied employees are the strongest assets and are the front-line promoters of value.

Participants' responses to questions that focused on the workforce identified a need for *value-focused* training. Participants discussed the need for value-focused training as opposed to just (any) 'training' referred in the Malcolm Baldrige model. This term referred to training focused on principles of delivering health care rooted in value. Participants widely varied in recommendations for the frequency of training and the number of resources used to develop or refine value-based behaviors. The frequency and type of training were dependent on the organization's culture and definitions of quality as indicated from their responses. Health-care organization leaders addressed the concern of balancing the use of resources for training. It was apparent for those that had not found strategies to reduce resource use, opined it may be necessary to 'bite-the-bullet' and allocate as much resources as necessary, especially if long-term returns have been considered.

Research-study participants believed in employee recognition to transform the health-care environment to an organization capable of meeting new health-care goals. Employee recognition as related by participants promotes a culture reinforcing appropriate behaviors and motivating the workforce. Although participants mentioned some of the workforce may possess an intrinsic motivation, employees still need rewards to improve the value of care for patients and for the organization, but is more effective when done after outcome measures are met. Participants had shared agreement that workforce engagement of the workforce that value can be increased for the patient. This employee engagement provides value to the organization in terms of the quality of work outcomes and encouragement of practices that optimizes organizational processes. Based on this data, the benefit of engagement of the workforce develops trust and motivates them, especially when employees are offered the opportunity to be part of the solution. Engagement as inferred by data analysis empowers employees to brainstorm collectively as needed to improve operational processes or patient's experience. Employee engagement in decision-making reduces the probability of strategy implementation failure, since employees are better informed. As a result, employees can function in a higher capacity to achieve organizational goals.

Discussion of Strategy Planning Findings

Strategy Planning in the Malcolm Baldrige model referred to leaders plans to prepare for its future sustenance. Preparation for the future is accomplished through development of short and long-term goals. The category addressed the necessary resources needed to realize the goals of such plans as well as methods of adapting plans, should circumstances change. Strategy Planning is the second element critical to a system's performance as defined by the Malcolm Baldrige model. Activities in this category involve creating well-defined plans designed for delivering quality to patients. Therefore, strategic plans also affect the operations and success of the organization. The importance of this category could be seen based on the number of efforts that participants offered that increases efficiency in processes and reduced overall costs. The number of strategies that leaders expressed to help promote improving value suggests there are no specific strategies leaders can emphasize to promote organizational success. It is possible no specific strategies have been identified, as the concept of value-based is relatively new, and organizations are implementing what they believe is best for the organization and its stakeholders. The lack of evidence-based strategies in this researcher's literature review specific to value-based health care can explain the element of concern participants expressed in terms of resource utilization in development and implementation of strategies. Responses can also be an indication of the lack of evidence-based practices; health-care leaders are currently using a compilation of their experience to facilitate longevity.

Reports by the Institute of Medicine, as discussed in the literature reviewed, highlighted the imperative of cost reduction as a contributor of sustainability of organizations. As interpreted from the research-study participants' responses and secondary data, participants seemed to heed the warning or at least made an effort to reduce costs. Research-study participants' responses highlighted strategies that increase value focused on clinical and operations processes. Health-care leader participants' responses reflected a commitment from leadership to ensure there is was no unnecessary waste through optimization of business processes.

Review of secondary data reflected that strategy planning was clearly inspired by the health-care organization's stated mission. Secondary data reflected a shared the mission to provide patient-centric care. Participants' responses indicate short-term goals are focused on evaluation of variations in costs and treatment plans, and the immediate money saving initiatives in the business, such as employee productivity, inventory control, and outsourcing of processes (mentioned by one participant). These responses are in alignment with some of the goals of the Affordable Care Act; making health care affordable to all, increasing access to care, accountability for health care actions, ensuring transparency in their services, and improving quality in the services delivered and outcomes of the care received (U.S. Department of Health and Human Services, 2013).

This research study's participants' responses indicated that employee and patient involvement is an immediate short-term goal that helps set the tone for continued value-based practices that permeates the culture of the organization in the long-term. Although responses indicated an integration of elements such as the employee and patients, resource use, and facilities management for optimal business process management, most of this research study's participants focused on strategies of sustainment to optimize processes to promote long-term success of the organization. The organizations' focus on sustainment strategies was understandable as many organizations are fearful of the financial sustenance from changes in the Medicare reimbursement for quality services.

Operation Focus

The Operation Focus category of the Malcolm Baldrige criteria refers to the approach health-care leaders use "to identify core competencies to achieve efficient and effective management of operations" (NIST, 2011, p. 21). The operation focus category examined the processes used to improve the organization's work system, meaning, how leaders ensure performance excellence as a reflection of value in its services. Such a focus, according to the Malcolm Baldrige model creates a competitive edge and, in the case of value-based health care, can promote efficiency. Data from participants' responses were supportive of findings from Trisolini et al. (2011) and Alexander and Hearld (2007), that organizations need to address activities in business or health-care operations to promote sustainability. Quality pioneers, including Donabedian and Deming, also stated the need to address the processes within an organization as means for quality improvement. Participants' responses supported these views; they saw the need for cost reduction and elimination of unnecessary waste as measures of efficiency. Participants offered the use of Lean and Six Sigma as ways to identify and reduce waste.

A focus on operations also included maximization of resources. Maximization of resources included employees working fully, performing tasks and job functions to the best quality and fullest capacity, using health-care related technology appropriately while not over-consuming resources. Crosby's (1992) research, highlighted the importance of limited deficiencies in the processes that deliver the product or service; this research study's participant responses indicated the need to eradicate processes within operations that do not contribute value to the patient or organization. From the secondary data source, this research study researcher observed a commitment to reduce activities and processes that produce little to no value to patients, especially through utilization of concepts such as Lean Six Sigma, and benchmarking to other organizations. Such commitment was evident in organizations including those not affected by Medicare's value-based health care. There is a unified commitment from the health-care organizations of accountability, responsibility, and dedication to delivering the best health care outcomes for patients. Health care's responsibility is also reflected in efforts to be more transparency of both healthcare and other, similar business operations to employees and patients.

Despite the relative newness of Medicare's program requirements, this research study's participants were aware of potential destructive financial effects of the concept on operations. Such awareness may be beneficial to leaders as they can be more prepared and have some type of forewarning about the implications of financial decisions. For example, one participant noted it is important for leaders to have the appropriate skill sets in leading the organization toward goal accomplishment. Without pertinent skills, there is higher risk of failure in accomplishing the task. There is also increased risk that staff will lose faith in leadership, which could lead to an unnecessary divide in organizational expectations that ultimately affects operations. Value-based health care is a relatively new concept; therefore, there may be many costly failures in terms of time and money to those entering this quality assurance arena. This is an area wherein preparedness will be beneficial to the success of the organization.

Discussion of Measurement, Analysis, and Knowledge Findings

This category examined how leaders integrate additional organizational to review and improves organizational performance and outcomes. The category also examined how facilitate decision-making and maintain a competitive position within health-care industry. Participants' responses in this category focused a need to assess the market and integrate outside information within operations. Benchmarking was a popular term used by participants to help evaluate practices within the organization. Although the Malcolm Baldrige model does not identify benchmarking as a specific element of business excellence, it is recognized that outside data should be reviewed (NIST, 2013). Performing a competitive analysis provides leaders with an idea of where the organization stands in relation to the same or similar health-care organization and industry leaders. Most participants agreed that benchmarking provides benefits; it was important to assess its applicability to the organization, rather than trying to imitate the competitor's processes. A few participants noted as an industry, leaders should look to other industries, such as the airline industry, to observe how those external to health-care organizations achieve excellence, improve quality standards or outcomes, and increase safety awareness for patients. While outside data was of significant value to the organization, the focus – according to the participants – should be if the organization is achieving the organization's quality metrics.

Results

This category examined how an organization performed in the rest of the Malcolm Baldrige categories in areas of process efficiency, preparedness, and operational effectiveness that impacts the outcomes for the customers. Performance in these areas is important to financial sustainability and accomplishment of strategic goals as a participant of Medicare's value-based health care program. Within this category, participants examined the organization's results according to a personal definition of success within the value-based program.

If value was viewed from a participant perspective, results are examined in areas of patient satisfaction, accountability, change in the patient's health status, costs for patient, and in the provision of appropriate treatment. From the perspective of value to the organization, results were examined in areas of accounts receivable, and accomplishment of business metrics.

Research Sub-Question Results

The insight gained from data collected, as discussed in the previous section, provided an understanding not only about the business strategies healthcare leaders use to increase the quality of care, but also identified business strategy gaps that could be filled. The interview data collected were reviewed further to develop an approach to find an answer for the research sub-question. The following section provides a detailed analysis.

The second research question sought to understand how organizations sustain a balance between increasing the value of care and lowering costs, while sustaining their financial growth. The previous discussion summarized the context about the dominant themes derived from interview data across the seven Baldrige categories. These research themes derived from participants' responses and secondary data to the main research question were further evaluated to understand the strategies that can be implemented to achieve the balance between operational cost, value of care, and financial growth.

Modified Malcolm Baldrige Model

From the research study analysis, data points toward an alternate form of the Malcolm Baldrige model that can be crafted and applied within health-care organizations. The model can be specific to value-based health care. Previously, organizations focused primarily on the businesses' financial bottom line and the Malcolm Baldrige model helped improve quality and performance excellence – with the intent to increase the competitive advantage and ultimately revenues. A proposed framework for the Malcolm Baldrige criteria could apply in this context of value-based health care where the focus is on earning maximum reimbursement, but with an equal focus on increasing the value of care for patients at significantly lower costs than previous operations (Figure 4).

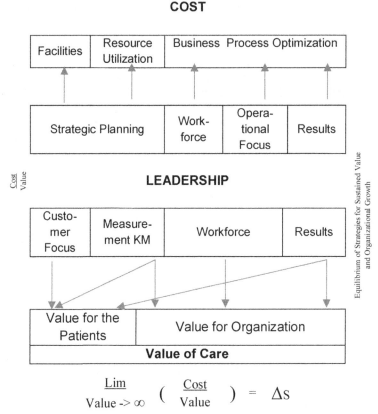

$$\underset{Value\ \to\ \infty}{Lim} \left(\frac{Cost}{Value} \right) = \Delta s$$

Figure 4 - Proposed Framework for Applied Malcolm Baldrige Criteria

(Where ΔS *(delta S)* is the deviation from the required state of financial equilibrium to sustain value and organizational growth)

The proposed framework was designed based on the synthesis of the thematic analysis of collected data. The framework suggests how various performance criteria can be focused on specific aspects of organizational development to attain the required balance between low cost operation, value of care, and financial growth. The model suggests while various performance criteria can be focused in specific segments, leadership continues to play the central role in increasing the value of care and consequently deriving results.

Leadership

In a non-value based model, sustained pursuit of quality remains the main driver for increased revenues and financial sustainability. In value-based health care, pursuit of quality is not merely for financial reasons but, for reasons of accountability and responsibility to deliver care appropriate, rooted in value, and at the lowest cost for the patient. Organizations achieve financial sustainability only when these elements are in alignment and is reflected in the organization's Medicare reimbursements.

For organizations to emphasize customer service, quality outcomes and efficiency are no longer options, but should be considered mandatory if organizations want to sustain the businesses' profitability. Leadership within this model is also the driving force to a sustained pursuit of quality and organizational longevity. The organizational leadership role is critical and central to defining values for a pay-for-performance culture and conveying these definitions to employees with a passion and clarity that permeates the organization and transforms the culture from volume (of services) to value (of health care provided to the patient). The messages of value-based care are mainly emphasizing the value of care delivered per dollars spent with best possible outcomes satisfactory to patient. The messages from leadership are not only communicated to employees, but also to the patients; leadership can have a better understanding of the patients' needs and expectations, as opposed to hypothesizing best methods that emphasize value.

A possible definition of financial growth for the health-care industry under the concept of value-based health care need to be redefined. The definition of financial growth can be accepted as the equilibrium of the strategies that can sustain a near-perfect cost value ratio for prolonged period of times, and allows the organization to grow in value of care is delivered in a longitudinal sense. To attain a near-perfect cost value ratio, the health-care organizational leadership would need to understand the components of both the value of care and operational costs.

Value of Care

Value of Care reflects how the research study participants (respondents) divided value of care into two perspectives; value as viewed from the patient's perspective and that of the combination of organizations and its employees' perspective. As a result, leaders need to understand both these perspectives so the right balance of strategies can be implemented. Responses from participants reflected that specific components of the Malcom Baldrige model are more applicable than others, depending on how value is perceived, and therefore will determine which strategies will produce the desired result. The findings from the data suggest that categories of customer and workforce focus, in addition to the results category, are more applicable in delivering value from the patient's perspective. Categories of workforce focus and results also overlap in delivering value for the organization. Measurement, knowledge, and analysis also directly impact the value for the organization.

Strategies within the Customer Focus category have a significant impact on the value for patients, especially if organizations fail to be reimbursed by Medicare, regardless of the value of the service to the patients. The strategies within the Workforce category also affect the value of care for patients as these health-care employees usually are those who make decisions regarding the delivery of care. These health-care employees are responsible for exuding behaviors rooted in value. Although organizations were customer-centric, clinical results were mainly measured from a financial perspective. In value-based health care, the results category needs to cater to outcomes primarily as meeting quality measure outcomes in specific clinical areas.

Strategies within the knowledge management, workforce and results criteria were also found to be of significant impact on the value of care for the organization. Responses gathered from the participants showed an affinity among workers to belong to an efficient value-based organization. It can be hypothesized that if health care organization leadership can be more definitive about the right values and instill them both in the workforce and the customer base, an organization could potentially attract high-quality, in-house experts – doctors, nurses, clinical specialists – who would be willing to associate with the organization, despite the higher earnings as a contractor.

Cost

The cost element refers to how organizations meet the national (Medicare influenced) mandate to reduce unnecessary wastage and improve quality at lower costs. Data revealed three major themes of lowering costs: Facilities, Resource Utilization, and Business and Process Optimization.

1. *Facilities.* Facilities refer to the necessity to form a mini-mergers or collaborations to form 'economies of scale.' This type of collaboration, according to participants, provides greater cost advantages to the organizations involved. Participants expressed this theme as part of the strategic planning category especially in terms of providing additional services they may not have offered

previously or attempted to achieve better quality
outcomes or achieve similar best practices within
the community.

2. *Resource Utilization.* Participants were very
   cognizant of resource use and most advised to
   reduce costs as strategic goals; it was important to
   prioritize goals or begin with issues most
   significant to the organization. However, though a
   critical component for reducing costs within the
   organization, participants thought sometimes a
   larger investment in resources is needed. Should
   this happen, participants voiced the long-term
   result should be reviewed before deciding to
   devote such resources to the initiative.
   Participants also shared it may be beneficial to
   form collaboration with organizations that can
   mentor organization leaders if there are not
   sufficient resources to develop suitable strategies.
   Participants expressed this theme as part of
   strategic planning, as leaders allocate resources
   to developing and implementing short and long
   term strategies.

3. *Business and Process Optimization.* Most of the
   responses to the interview questions elicited a
   response to optimize business-process, cost
   savings passed along to patients. There is the
   potential for the volume of patients to decrease.
   Leaders seem to be proactive in reducing defects,
   redundant steps, or non-value-added activities that
   lead to a highly functioning system delivering high
   quality services. The components of workforce,

results, operation, and measurement and analysis focused on business and process optimization.

The framework discussed above deviates from the typical health care organization models in that it does not consider immediate financial gains as a measure of excellence. The Malcolm Baldridge model proposes to deploy a strong leadership, and financial analysis as a central agent, that focuses solely on maintaining the cost-to-value ratio and steer the organization on a path of longitudinal growth. Aligned with the intended vision of Medicare's value-based program, application of the Malcolm Baldridge model could provide the required balance between maintaining low cost operations, high value of care, and longitudinal financial growth for health providers.

Although a qualitative methodology was deemed appropriate for this research, a quantitative study may have allowed more objectivity and a larger number of participants. Methods to increase validity and reliability pertaining to this research study included use of semi-structured interview questionnaire, which increased the opportunity for unbiased findings, as well as allowing participants to check the transcripts to ensure accuracy of information captured.

A qualitative methodology limited the study such that findings from qualitative studies cannot be generalized beyond the participants of this research. As a result, there is no guarantee the outcomes of this research study are transferable to other leaders of health-care organizations. It is anticipated these participants share similar goals in finding the necessary balance between financial viability and delivering a high quality of care. This study followed a systematic and methodological design and offered insight to approaches taken to conduct the research. This transparency, according to Swanson and Holton (2005), will allow other researchers to deem whether the design is consistent with the research's purposes, method, and analysis.

The study was inclusive of organizations across the United States. There may have be additional factors such as geographic location, population, size, and ownership that influenced responses to the interview questions and as such may have provided an inconsistent guideline to strategies that work best in achieving the goals of value-based health care.

Implications

The outcomes of this qualitative study led to a deeper understanding of value-based, health care and an overview of the business practices that can be implemented. The most important outcome was the recognition of business practices that can lead to improvement in the quality and value of care, accountability of practices and services, and a holistic transformation of the healthcare system.

First, the study implied the best practices are dependent on the organization's definition of quality, value, and success in the program. One of the main focuses of value-based health care is the patient, the other being cost. The study indicated value must be recognized from a three-dimensional perspective concept; that of value as viewed by the patient, the organization, and the organization's perceived perspective of value to the patient. Therefore, leaders need to examine the components of value-based care and the influence of these elements on quality improvement and performance excellence. Leaders can adopt or examine the strategies presented in this study for suitability for its use in accomplishing organizational goals.

Second, the study showed organizations with limited access to resources should not be as concerned about the organization's ability to improve value of care and outcomes. Increased collaborative efforts between organizations can ease the burden of change. Collaborative efforts between other health-care facilities not only maximize resource use, but increases health-care accountability through cost containment and improved quality outcomes for patients. Collaborative efforts help organizations who are unable to meet clinical quality outcome measures. Through collaboration, organizations can do what is right for patients to increase the patient's quality of life.

This qualitative case study used the Malcolm Baldrige Criteria for Performance Excellence model and presented a gap between the conceptual value-based healthcare model and its implementation. Medicare designed the program with the idea of improving value for its beneficiaries and reducing the unnecessary costs associated with health-care services that is critical to improvement of the entire system. The problem is a detailed guide to delivering value-based, health care is lacking. Implications of this study suggest the gap could be filled by implementing the modified Malcolm Baldrige model for performance excellence. This modified model provides equilibrium of strategies for sustained value delivered to patients and organizational growth. The proposed framework based on the modified Malcolm Baldrige criteria may allow the leadership of health-care organizations to adopt strategies that can implement the value-based Medicare program and achieve the intended results – better medical care – of the program. Medicare officials expect leaders to improve their health-care organization's efficiency, reduce costs, and increase the value of care. It is important that health-care organization leaders are aware of the strategies to help facilitate their success in Medicare's program to remain financially viable. Although these reforms are major prospects for improvement in payment and the delivery of care, it is not a complete solution to reducing costs and increasing quality.

The study further indicated it is possible for organizations to achieve the balance between costs, value, and finances. Additional attention needs to be directed at the definition of financial success in value-based health care. Financial growth in value-based health care should be considered based on the organization's ability to sustain the cost-value ratio over the long term instead of from its traditional perspective of profitability.

Recommendations for Future Research

The outcomes of this study addressed the research questions presented in Chapter 1. Use of the Malcolm Baldrige Criteria framework answered the research questions in this study. The analysis and discussion of findings with the implications confirmed the Malcolm Baldrige Criteria for Performance Excellence is an appropriate quality improvement tool whose underlying foundations of total quality management can be used as a theoretical framework for facilitating success in Medicare's value-based health care program.

The following recommendations support future use of the Baldrige Criteria for Performance Excellence in value-based health care.

1. Future research can further refine interview questions and examine categories of the Malcolm Baldrige Criteria for Health Care separately to identify the best strategies with possible implications applied to facilitate success in value-based health care.
2. This study can be replicated to examine best strategies (different levels of ownership in health care) to further narrow strategies specific to non-profit, for-profit, and government-owned facilities.
3. This study can be used in future studies based on the Malcolm Baldrige criteria to determine best strategies for success in specific areas such as improvement in customer satisfaction or in operation efficiency.
4. A study can be conducted on best strategies specific to accomplishing goals as these strategies may vary according to long- or short-term goals.
5. Future research can use this study's strategies to assess long-term impact on financial sustainability on organizations.
6. A future study can examine the differences in best business practices as identified by front-line staff, middle managers, and upper management.
7. This study can be replicated to determine if the Malcolm Baldrige Criteria for Performance Excellence is applicable to Veteran's Affairs Hospitals (cost of health care is not a critical factor).

8. A similar study could be conducted to compare the impact of reimbursement amounts for organizations using business strategies as a guideline versus organizations without.
9. A study can be conducted to examine impacts of patient education and engagement on clinical outcomes.

REFERENCES

Alexander, J. A., & Hearld, L. R. (2009). What can we learn from quality improvement research? A critical review of research methods. *Medical Care Research and Review, 66*, 235-271. doi:10.1177/1077558708330424.

Alexander, J. A., Hearld, L. R., Jiang, H. J., & Fraser, I. (2007). Increasing the relevance of research to health care managers: Hospital CEO imperatives for improving quality and lowering costs. *Health Care Management Review, 32*, 150-159.

American Society of Quality. (2013). *How do you define quality?* Retrieved from http://asq.org/blog/2013/01/how-do-you-define-quality/

Asubonteng, P., McCleary, K. J., & Munchus, G. (1996). The evolution of quality in the US health-care industry: An old wine in a new bottle. *International Journal of Health Care Quality Assurance, 9*(3), 11-19.

Badri, M. A., Selim, H., Alshare, K., Grandon, E. E., Younis, H., & Abdulla, M. (2006). The Baldrige education criteria for performance excellence framework: Empirical test and validation. *International Journal of Quality and Reliability Management, 23*, 1118-1157.

Baicker, K., & Chandra, A. (2009). Medicare spending, the physician workforce, and beneficiaries' quality of care. *Health Affairs (Millwood), 28*(1), 119-23.

Baxter, P., & Jack, S. (2008). Qualitative case study methodology: Study design and implementation for novice researchers. *The Qualitative Report, 13*, 544-559. Retrieved from http://www.nova.edu/ssss/QR/QR13-4/baxter.pdf

Beauvais, B., & Wells, R. (2006). Does money really matter? A review of the literature on the relationships between healthcare organization finances and quality. *Hospital Topics, 84*(2), 20-29.

Bell, R. R., & Elkins, S. A. (2004). A balanced scorecard for leaders: Implications of the Malcolm Baldrige National Quality Award criteria. *SAM Advanced Management Journal, 69*(1), 12-17.

Berwick, D. M. (2002). A user's manual for the IOM's 'Quality Chasm' report. *Health Affairs, 21*(3), 80-90. doi:10.1377/hlthaff.21.3.80

Berwick, D. M., & Hackbarth, A. D. (2012). Eliminating waste in US health care. *JAMA: The Journal of the American Medical Association, 307*, 1513-1516.

Berwick, D. M., Nolan, T. W., & Whittington, J. (2008). The triple aim: Care, health, and cost. *Health Affairs, 27*, 759-769.

Blumenthal, D., & Kilo, C. M. (1998). A report card on continuous quality improvement. *Milbank Quarterly, 76*, 625-648.

Borden, W. B., & Blustein, J. (2012). Valuing improvement in value-based purchasing. *Circulation: Cardiovascular Quality and Outcomes, 5*, 163-170.

Braveman, P. A., Cubbin, C., Egerter, S., Williams, D. R., & Pamuk, E. (2010). Socioeconomic disparities in health in the United States: What the patterns tell us. *Journal Information, 100*, Suppl 1, S186-196. doi:10.2105/AJPH.2009.166082

Bryman, A. (2008). *Social research methods* (3rd ed.). New York, NY: Oxford University Press.

Bush, H. (2012). Health care's costliest. *Hospital Health Network, 86*(9), 30-34, 36.

Bush, R. W. (2007). Reducing waste in US health-care systems. *JAMA: The Journal of the American Medical Association, 297*, 871-874.

Buttell, P., Hendler, R., & Daley, J. (2008). *Quality in healthcare: concepts and practice. The business of healthcare.* Westport, CT: Praeger. Retrieved from http://healthcarecollaboration.com/docs/quality_buttell.pdf

Centers for Medicare and Medicaid Services. (2011). *Hospital value-based purchasing program. Fact sheet.* Retrieved from http://www.cms.gov/Hospital-Value-Based-Purchasing

Centers for Medicare and Medicaid Services. (2012). *Hospital quality initiative.* Retrieved from http://www.cms.gov/Medicare/Quality-Initiatives-Patient-Assessment-Instruments/HospitalQualityInits/index.html?redirect=/HospitalQualityInits/

Centers for Medicare and Medicaid Services. (2013). *HCAHPS: Patients' perspectives of care survey.* Retrieved from http://www.cms.gov/Medicare/Quality-Initiatives-Patient-Assessment-Instruments/HospitalQualityInits/HospitalHCAHPS.html

Champy, J., & Greenspun, H. (2010). *Reengineering health care: A manifesto for radically rethinking health care delivery.* Upper Saddle River, NJ: Pearson.

Chassin, M. R., & Galvin, R. W. (1998). The urgent need to improve health care quality. *JAMA: The Journal of the American Medical Association, 280*, 1000-1005.

Chassin, M. R., & Loeb, J. M. (2011). The ongoing quality improvement journey: Next stop, high reliability. *Health Affairs, 30*, 559-568.

Chassin, M. R., Loeb, J. M., Schmaltz, S. P., & Wachter, R. M. (2010). Accountability measures—using measurement to promote quality improvement. *New England Journal of Medicine, 363*, 683-688.

Chodhury, J. S., Kapur, A., Saxena, S. B., & Topdjian, J. (2011). *Unlocking value in healthcare transformation through collaboration.* Retrieved from http://www.booz.com/media/file/Unlocking_Value_in_Healthcare.pdf

Chrusciel, D., & Field, D. W. (2003). From critical success factors into criteria for performance excellence–an organizational change strategy. *Journal of Industrial Technology, 19*(4), 1-11.

Clancy, C. (2005). *AHRQ Summit—Improving health care quality for all Americans: The quality challenge.* Agency for Healthcare Research and Quality (AHRQ). U.S. Department of Health and Human Services. Retrieved from http://www.ahrq.gov/legacy/qual/qsummit/qsummit1.htm

Cohen, D. J., & Crabtree, B. F. (2008). Evaluative criteria for qualitative research in health care: Controversies and recommendations. *Annals of Family Medicine, 6*, 331-339. doi:10.1370/afm.818

Committee on Quality of Health Care in America, Institute of Medicine. (2011).*Crossing the quality chasm: A new health system for the 21st century.* Washington, DC: National Academy Press. Retrieved from http://www.nap.edu/openbook.php?isbn=0309072808

Cooper, A., Reeves, S., & Levinson, W. (2008). An introduction to reading and appraising qualitative research. *British Medical Journal, 337*. doi:10.1136/bmj.a288

Cooper, C. R., & Schindler, P. S. (2011). *Business research methods* (11th ed.). Boston, MA: McGraw-Hill.

Corbin, J., & Strauss, A. L. (2007). *Basics of qualitative research. Techniques and procedures for developing grounded theory* (3rd ed.). Thousand Oaks, CA: Sage.

Creswell, J. W. (2007). *Qualitative, inquiry and research design: Choosing among five approaches* (2nd ed.). Thousand Oaks, CA: Sage.

Creswell, J. W. (2009). *Research design: Qualitative, quantitative, and mixed methods approaches* (3rd ed.). Thousand Oaks, CA: Sage.

Cromwell, J., Trisolini, M. G., Pope, G. C., Mitchell, J. B., & Greenwald, L. M. (Eds.).(2011). *Pay-for-performance in health care: Methods and approaches.* Retrieved from https://www.rti.org/pubs/bk-0002-1103-mitchell.pdf

Crosby, P. B. (1992). *Completeness: Quality for the twenty-first century.* London, England: Penguin.

Curkovic, S., Melnyk, S., Calantone, R., & Handfield, R. (2000). Validating the Malcolm Baldrige national quality award framework through structural equation modeling. *International Journal of Production Research, 38,* 765-791. doi:10.1080/002075400189149

Dahlgaard, J. J., Pettersen, J., & Dahlgaard-Park, S. M. (2011). Quality and lean health care: A system for assessing and improving the health of healthcare organisations. *Total Quality Management and Business Excellence, 22,* 673-689.

DeBaylo, P. W. (1999). Ten reasons why the Baldrige model works. *Journal for Quality and Participation, 22,* 24-29.

Dellana, S. A., & Hauser, R. D. (1999). Toward defining the quality culture. *Engineering Management Journal-Rolla, 11,* 11-16.

Denzin, N. K., & Lincoln, Y. S. (1998). *Strategies of qualitative inquiry.* Thousand Oaks, CA: Sage.

Denzin, N. K., & Lincoln, Y. S. (Eds.). (2005). *The Sage handbook of qualitative research.* Thousand Oaks, CA: Sage.

Donabedian, A. (2005). Evaluating the quality of medical care. *Milbank Quarterly, 83,* 691-729. doi:10.1111/j.1468-0009.2005.00397.x

Donaldson, M. S., & Mohr, J. J. (2000). *Improvement and innovation in health care microsystems.* A Technical Report for the Institute of Medicine Committee on the Quality of Health Care in America. Princeton: Robert Wood Johnson Foundation.

Eijkenaar, F. (2012). Pay-for-performance in health care: An international overview of initiatives. *Medical Care Research and Review, 69,* 251-276.

Eisenhardt, K. M. (1989). Building theories from case study research. *Academy of Management Review, 14,* 532-550.

Epstein, A. M. (2006). Paying for performance in the United States and abroad. *New England Journal of Medicine, 355,* 406-408.

Evans, I., Thornton, H., Chalmers, I., & Glasziou, P. (2011). *Testing treatments: Better research for better healthcare* (2nd ed.). London, England: Pinter & Martin.

Evans, J. R., & Jack, E. P. (2003). Validating key results linkages in the Baldrige performance excellence model. *Quality Management Journal, 10*(2), 7-24.

Fening, F. A., Pesakovic, G., & Amaria, P. (2008). Relationship between quality management practices and the performance of small and medium size enterprises (SMEs) in Ghana. *International Journal of Quality and Reliability Management, 25,* 694-708.

Fenter, T. C., & Lewis, S. J. (2008). Pay-for-performance initiatives. *Journal of Managed Care Pharmacy, 14*(6), S12-S15.

Flynn, B. B., & Saladin, B. (2001). Further evidence on the validity of the theoretical models underlying the Baldrige criteria. *Journal of Operations Management, 19,* 617–652.

Foster, T. C., Johnson, J. K., Nelson, E. C., & Batalden, P. B. (2007). Using a Malcolm Baldrige framework to understand high-performing clinical microsystems. *Quality and Safety in Health Care, 16,* 334-341.

Fotopoulos, C. B., & Psomas, E. L. (2009). The impact of "soft" and "hard" TQM elements on quality management results, *International Journal of Quality and Reliability Management, 26,* 150-163.

Future Directions for the National Healthcare Quality and Disparities Reports. (2010). Institute of Medicine. Retrieved from http://iom.edu/Reports.aspx?Topic1={DE49DD61-623A-438F-932B-6921E7BE9F6A}&Topic2={F41F0DA6-1C6F-4B9A-B1AF-A4DD17336E54}&page=2

Gall, M. D., Borg, W. R., & Gall, J. P. (2002). *An introduction to educational research* (8th ed.). Thousand Oaks, CA: Sage.

Gamm, L. D., Hutchison, L. L., Dabney, B. J., & Dorsey, A. (2003). Rural healthy people. Public health rural health priorities in America: Where you stand depends on where you sit. *The Journal of Rural Health, 19,* 209-213.

Gangeness, J., & Yurkovich, E. (2006). Revisiting case study as a nursing research design. *Nurse Researcher, 13*(4), 7-18.

Gibbert, M., Ruigrok, W., & Wicki, B. (2008). What passes as a rigorous case study? *Strategic Management Journal, 29,* 1465-1474.

Golafshani, N. (2003). Understanding reliability and validity in qualitative research. *The Qualitative Report, 8,* 597-607. Retrieved from http://www.nova.edu/ssss/QR/QR8-4/golafshani.pdf

Goonan, K. J., & Muzikowski, J. (2008). Baldrige: Myths and realities. *Hospitals and Health Networks, 82,* 84-85.

Goulding, C. (2005). Grounded theory, ethnography, and phenomenology: A comparative analysis of three qualitative strategies for marketing research. *European Journal of Marketing, 39,* 294-308.

Green, J., & Thorogood, N. (2009). *Qualitative methods for health research.* London, England: Sage.

Greene, S. E., & Nash, D. B. (2009). Pay-for-performance: An overview of the literature. *American Journal of Medical Quality, 24,* 140-163.

Guest, G., Bunce, A., & Johnson, L. (2006). How many interviews are enough? An experiment with data saturation and variability. *Field Methods, 18*(1), 59-82.

Hackman, J. R., & Wageman, R. (1995). Total quality management: Empirical, conceptual, and practical issues. *Administrative Science Quarterly, 40,* 309-342.

Han, S. B., Chen, S. K., Ebrahimpour, M., & Sodhi, M. S. (2001). A conceptual QFD planning model. *International Journal of Quality and Reliability Management, 18,* 796-812.

Hancock, D. R., & Algozzine, B. (2006). *Doing case study research. A practical guide for beginning researchers.* New York, NY: Teachers College Press.

Handfield, R. B., & Ghosh, S. (1995). An empirical test of linkages between the Baldrige criteria and financial performance. In *Proceedings of the Decision Sciences Institute* (Vol. 3, pp. 1713-1715). Boston, MA: Decision Sciences Institute.

Hartman, M., Martin, A. B., Benson, J., & Catlin, A. (2013). National health spending in 2011: Overall growth remains low, but some payers and services show signs of acceleration. *Health Affairs (Millwood), 32*(1), 87-99. doi:10.1377/hlthaff.2012.1206

Heffner, J. E., Mularski, R. A., & Calverley, P. M. (2010). COPD Performance measures: Missing opportunities for improving care. *CHEST Journal, 137,* 1181-1189.

Hellsten, U., & Klefsjö, B. (2000). TQM as a management system consisting of values, techniques and tools. *The TQM Magazine, 12,* 238-244.

Hermer, L. D., & Brody, H. (2010). Defensive medicine, cost containment, and reform. *Journal of General Internal Medicine, 25,* 470-478.

Hibbard, J., & Sofaer, S. (2010). *Best practices in public reporting no. 1: How to effectively present health care performance data to consumers.* Agency for Healthcare Research and Quality. Retrieved from http://www.ahrq.gov/legacy/qual/pubrptguide1.htm

Hines, P. A., & Yu, K. M. (2009). The changing reimbursement landscape: Nurses' role in quality and operational excellence. *Nurse Economics Journal, 27*(1), 1-7.

Hospital Value-Based Purchasing Program. (2011). *Fact sheet.* Department of Health and Human Services. Centers for Medicare and Medicaid Services. Retrieved from http://www.cms.gov/Hospital-Value-Based-Purchasing

Institute of Medicine. (2010). *Future directions for the national healthcare quality and disparities reports.* Retrieved from http://iom.edu/Reports.aspx?Topic1={DE49DD61-623A-438F-932B-6921E7BE9F6A}&Topic2={F41F0DA6-1C6F-4B9A-B1AF-A4DD17336E54}&page=2

Institute of Medicine. (2012). *For the public's health, investing in a healthier future.* Retrieved from http://www.iom.edu/Reports/2012/For-the-Publics-Health-Investing-in-a-Healthier-Future.aspx

Jacob, R. A., Madu, C. N., & Tang, C. (2012). Financial performance of Baldrige award winners: A review and synthesis. *The International Journal of Quality and Reliability Management, 29,* 233-240. doi:http://dx.doi.org/10.1108/02656711211199937

Jayamaha, N. P., Grigg, N. P., & Mann, R. S. (2008). Empirical validity of Baldrige criteria: New Zealand evidence. *International Journal of Quality and Reliability Management, 25,* 477-493.

Jencks, S. F., Williams, M. V., & Coleman, E. A. (2009). Rehospitalizations among patients in the Medicare fee-for-service program. *New England Journal of Medicine, 360,* 1418-1428.

Johnson, R. B. (1997). Examining the validity structure of qualitative research. *Education, 118,* 282-292.

Jones, N., Jones, S. L., & Miller, N. A. (2004). The Medicare Health Outcomes Survey program: Overview, context, and near-term prospects. *Health and Quality of Life Outcomes, 2*(1), 33-35.

Juran, J. M. (1993). Made in USA: A renaissance in quality. *Harvard Business Review, 71*(4), 42-47.

Khamalah, J. N., & Lingaraj, B. P. (2007). TQM in the service sector: A survey of small businesses. *Total Quality Management, 18,* 973-982.

Kohn, L. T., Corrigan, J. M., & Donaldson, M. S. (2001). Crossing the quality chasm: A new health system for the 21st century. *Washington, DC: Committee on Quality of Health Care in America, Institute of Medicine.*

Kohn, L. T., Corrigan, J. M., & Donaldson, M. S. (Eds.). (2000). *To err is human. Building a safer health system.* Washington, DC: National Academy Press.

Komashie, A., Mousavi, A., & Gore, J. (2007). Quality management in healthcare and industry: A comparative review and emerging themes. *Journal of Management History, 13,* 359-370.

Korenstein, D., Falk, R., Howell, E. A., Bishop, T., & Keyhani, S. (2012). Overuse of health-care services in the United States: An understudied problem. *Archives of Internal Medicine, 172,* 171-179.

Kumar, S., Ghildayal, N. S., & Shah, R. N. (2011). Examining quality and efficiency of the US healthcare system. *International Journal of Health Care Quality Assurance, 24,* 366-388.

Kumar, V., Choisne, F., de Grosbois, D., & Kumar, U. (2009). Impact of TQM on company's performance. *International Journal of Quality and Reliability*

Management, 26(1), 23-37.

Landrigan, C. P., Parry, G. J., Bones, C. B., Hackbarth, A. D., Goldmann, D. A., & Sharek, P. J. (2010). Temporal trends in rates of patient harm resulting from medical care. *New England Journal of Medicine, 363,* 2124-2134.

Leape, L. L., & Berwick, D. M. (2005). Five years after "To Err is Human". *JAMA: The Journal of the American Medical Association, 293,* 2384-2390.

Leape, L., Berwick, D., Clancy, C., Conway, J., Gluck, P., Guest, J.,... Isaac, T. (2009). Transforming healthcare: A safety imperative. *Quality and Safety in Health Care, 18,* 424-428.

Lenka, U., & Suar, D. (2008). A holistic model of total quality management in services. *The Icfaian Journal of Management Research, 7*(3), 56-72.

Lincoln, Y. S., & Guba, E. (1985). *Naturalistic inquiry.* Thousand Oaks, CA: Sage.

Linn, S. T., Guralnik, J. M., & Patel, K. V. (2010). Disparities in influenza vaccine coverage in the United States, 2008. *Journal of the American Geriatrics Society, 58,* 1333-1340.

Loomba, A. P., & Johannessen, T. B. (1997). Malcolm Baldrige National Quality Award: critical issues and inherent values. *Benchmarking for Quality Management and Technology, 4*(1), 59-77.

Lowder, B. (2009). *Choosing a methodology for entrepreneurial research: A case for qualitative research in the study of entrepreneurial success factors.* Retrieved from http://papers.ssrn.com/sol3/papers.cfm?abstract_id=1411914

Luce, J. M., Bindman, A. B., & Lee, P. R. (1994). A brief history of health care quality assessment and improvement in the United States. *Western Journal of Medicine, 160,* 263-273.

Lukas, C. V., Holmes, S. K., Cohen, A. B., Restuccia, J., Cramer, I. E., Shwartz, M., & Charns, M. P. (2007). Transformational change in health-care systems: an organizational model. *Health Care Management Review, 32*(4), 309-320.

Mahapatra, S. S., & Khan, M. S. (2006). Current practices of TQM implementation and future trend. *Industrial Engineering Journal, 35*(5), 28-33.

Mant, J. (2001). Process versus outcome indicators in the assessment of quality of health care. *International Journal for Quality in Health Care, 13,* 475-480.

Marmor, T., & Oberlander, J. (2011). The patchwork: Health reform, American style. *Social Science and Medicine, 72*(2), 125-131.

Marmor, T., Oberlander, J., & White, J. (2009). The Obama administration's options for health care cost control: Hope versus reality. *Annals of Internal Medicine, 150,* 485-489.

Marshall, M. N. (1996). Sampling for qualitative research. *Family Practice, 13,* 522-526.

Mason, M. (2010, August). Sample size and saturation in PhD studies using qualitative interviews. In *Forum Qualitative Sozial for Schung/Forum: Qualitative Social Research* (Vol. 11, No. 3).

Maxwell, J. A. (1992). Understanding validity in qualitative research. *Harvard Educational Review, 62,* 279-300.

McIntyre, D., Rogers, L., & Heier, E. J. (2001). Overview, history, and objectives of performance measurement. *Health Care Financing Review, 22*(3), 7-22.

McWilliams, J. M., Meara, E., Zaslavsky, A. M., & Ayanian, J. Z. (2009). Differences in control of cardiovascular disease and diabetes by race, ethnicity, and education: US trends from 1999 to 2006 and effects of Medicare coverage. *Annals of Internal Medicine, 150,* 505-515.

Medicare Payment Advisory Commission.(2013). *Medicare and the healthcare delivery system.* Report to Congress. Retrieved from http://www.medpac.gov/documents/Jun13_EntireReport.pdf

Mehrotra, A., Damberg, C. L., Sorbero, M. E., & Teleki, S. S. (2009). Pay-for-performance in the hospital setting: What is the state of the evidence? *American Journal of Medical Quality, 24*(1), 19-28.

Merriam, S. B. (1998).*Qualitative research and case study applications in education.* San Francisco, CA: Jossey-Bass.

Miles, M., & Huberman, A. (1994). *Qualitative data analysis* (2nd ed.). Thousand Oaks, CA: Sage.

Mohammad, M., Mann, R., Grigg, N., & Wagner, J. P. (2011). Business Excellence Model: An overarching framework for managing and aligning multiple organisational improvement initiatives. *Total Quality Management and Business Excellence, 22*, 1213-1236.

Montgomery, D. C. (2010). A modern framework for achieving enterprise excellence. *International Journal of Lean Six Sigma, 1*(1), 56-65.

Muenning, P. A., & Glied, S. A. (2010). What changes in survival rates tell us about US health care. *Health Affairs, 29*, 2105-2113.

Nahed, B. V., Babu, M. A., Smith, T. R., & Heary, R. F. (2012). Malpractice liability and defensive medicine: A national survey of neurosurgeons. (*PLoS) Public Library of Science One, 7*(6), e39237. doi:10.1371/journal.pone.0039237.

National Institutes of Health. (1999). *Health disparities defined.* Retrieved from http://crchd.cancer.gov/disparities/defined.html

National Institutes of Health. (2008). *Baldrige national quality program. The Malcolm Baldrige National Quality Improvement Act of 1987-Public Law 100-107.* Retrieved from http://www.quality.nist.gov/Improvement_Act.html

National Institutes of Health. (2010). *Baldrige national quality program. Healthcare criteria for performance excellence.* Retrieved from www.baldrige.nist.gov\

National Institutes of Health. (2013). *Health care criteria for performance excellence.* Retrieved from http://www.nist.gov/baldrige/publications/upload/Category_and_Item_Commentary_HC.pdf

Nelson, E. C., Batalden, P. B, Homa, K., Godfrey, M. M., Campbell, C., Headrick, L. A.,.. Wasson, J. H. (2003). Microsystems in health care: Part 2. Creating a rich information environment. *Joint Commission Journal Quality Safety, 29*(1), 5–15.

Nelson, M. L., & Quintana, S. M. (2005). Qualitative clinical research with children and adolescents. *Journal of Clinical Child and Adolescent Psychology, 34*, 344-356.

Nielsen, D. (2005). Baldrige award's blueprint for excellence. *AHA News, 41*(4), 5. Retrieved from http://www.ahanews.com/ahanews/

Orszag, P. R. (2008). *The overuse, underuse, and misuse of health care.* Statement before the Committee on Finance, US Senate. Retrieved from http://www.cbo.gov/publication/41718

Osborne, J. W. (1994). Some similarities and differences among phenomenological and other methods of psychological qualitative research. *Canadian Psychology/Psychologie Canadienne, 35*(2), 167-170.

Pannirselvam, G. P., & Ferguson, L. A. (2001). A study of the relationships between the Baldrige categories. *International Journal of Quality and Reliability Management, 18*(1), 14-37.

Patient Protection and Affordable Care Act, Pub. L. No. 111-148, §2702, 124 Stat. 119, 318-319 (2010).

Patton, M. Q. (2002). Two decades of developments in qualitative inquiry: A personal, experiential perspective. *Qualitative Social Work, 1*, 261-283.

Peterson, C. L., & Burton, R. (2011). *US health care spending: Comparison with other OECD countries.* Federal Publications. Cornell University. Retrieved from http://digitalcommons.ilr.cornell.edu/cgi/viewcontent.cgi?article=1316&context =key_workplace

Pettypiece, S., & Armour, S. (2013). *Billion-dollar hospital bonuses not seen improving health.* Retrieved from http://www.bloomberg.com/news/2013-01-25/billion-dollar-hospital-bonuses-not-seen-improving-health.html

Polkinghorne, D. E. (2005). Language and meaning: Data collection in qualitative research. *Journal of Counseling Psychology, 52,* 137-140.

Pope, C., & Mays, N. (2008). *Qualitative research in health care* (3rd ed.). Boston, MA: Blackwell.

Porter, L. J., & Parker, A. J. (1993). Total Quality Management the critical success factors. *Total Quality Management, 4*(3), 13-22.

Porter, M. E. (2009). A strategy for health-care reform-toward a value-based system. *The New England Journal of Medicine, 361,* 109-112. doi:10.1056/NEJMp0904131.

Porter, M. E. (2010). What is value in health care? *The New England Journal of Medicine, 363,* 277-281. doi:http://dx.doi.org/10.1056/NEJMp1011024

Prajogo, D. I., & Brown, A. (2004). The relationship between TQM practices and quality performance and the role of formal TQM programs: An Australian empirical study. *Quality Management Journal, 11,* 31–43.

Prendergast, C. (1999). The provision of incentives in firms. *Journal of Economic Literature, 37*(1), 7-63.

Quinn, S. C., Kumar, S., Freimuth, V. S., Musa, D., Casteneda-Angarita, N., & Kidwell, K. (2011). Racial disparities in exposure, susceptibility, and access to health care in the US H1N1 influenza pandemic. *American Journal of Public Health, 101,* 285-293. doi:10.2105/AJPH.2009.188029.

Reason, P., & Rowan, J. (1981). *Human inquiry: A sourcebook of new paradigm research.* London, England: John Wiley & Sons.

Reinier, K., Thomas, E., Andrusiek, D. L., Aufderheide, T. P., Brooks, S. C., Callaway, C. W.,... Chugh, S. S. (2011). Socioeconomic status and incidence of sudden cardiac arrest. *Canadian Medical Association Journal, 183,* 1705-1712.

Repenning, N. P., & Sterman, J. D. (2001). Nobody ever gets credit for fixing problems that never happened. *California Management Review, 43*(4), 64-88.

Ricondo, I., & Viles, E. (2005). Six Sigma and its link to TQM, BPR, Lean and the learning organisation. *International Journal of Six Sigma and Competitive Advantage, 1,* 323-354.

Ridder, H. G., Hoon, C., & McCandless, A. (2009). The theoretical contribution of case study research to the field of strategy and management. *Research Methodology in Strategy and Management, 5,* 137-175.

Riege, A. M. (2003). Validity and reliability tests in case study research: a literature review with "hands-on" applications for each research phase. *Qualitative Market Research: An International Journal, 6*(2), 75-86.

Robinson, J. C. (2001). Theory and practice in the design of physician payment incentives. *Milbank Quarterly, 79,* 149-177.

Robson, C. (2002). *Real world research: A resource for social scientists and practitioner-researchers* (Vol. 2). Oxford, England: Blackwell.

Roland, M. (2012). Pay-for-performance: Not a magic bullet. *Annals of Internal Medicine, 157,* 912-913.

Rosenthal, M. B., & Frank, R. G. (2006). What is the empirical basis for paying for quality in health care? *Medical Care Research and Review, 63,* 135-157.

Sadikoglu, E. (2008). Total quality management practices and performance. *The Business Review, Cambridge, 10*(2), 60-68.

Salaheldin, S. I. (2009). Critical success factors for TQM implementation and their impact on performance of SMEs. *International Journal of Productivity and Performance Management, 58*, 215-237.

Samson, D., & Terziovski, M. (1999). The relationship between total quality management practices and operational performance. *Journal of Operations Management, 17*, 393-409.

Schoen, C. (2013). *Confronting costs: Stabilizing U.S. health spending while moving toward a high performance health-care system.* Retrieved from http://www.commonwealthfund.org/Publications/Fund-Reports/2013/Jan/Confronting-Costs.aspx?page=all#citation

Sheingold, S. H., & Lied, T. R. (2001). An overview: The future of plan performance measurement. *Health Care Financing Review, 22*(3), 1-6.

Sherwood, G. (2012). *Driving forces for quality and safety: Changing mindsets to improve health care. Quality and safety in nursing: A competency approach to improving outcomes.* Ames, IA: John Wiley & Sons.

Shewhart, W. A. (1931). *Economic control of quality of manufactured product.* Milwaukee, WI: Asq Press.

Sila, I. (2007). Examining the effects of contextual factors on TQM and performance through the lens of organizational theories: An empirical study. *Journal of Operations Management, 25*(1), 83-109.

Skrinjar, R., Bosilj-Vukšic, V., & Indihar-Štemberger, M. (2008). The impact of business process orientation on financial and non-financial performance. *Business Process Management Journal, 14*, 738-754.

Soy, S. K. (1997). *The case study as a research method.* Unpublished paper, University of Texas at Austin. Retrieved from http://www.ischool.utexas.edu/~ssoy/usesusers/l391d1b.htm.

Spencer, B. A. (1994). Models of organization and total quality management: a comparison and critical evaluation. *Academy of Management Review, 19*, 446-471.

Squires, D. A. (2012). Issues in international health policy: explaining high health-care spending in the United States: an international comparison of supply, utilization, prices, and quality. *Issue brief (Commonwealth Fund), 10*, 1.

Stake, R. (1995*). The art of case study research.* Thousand Oaks, CA: Sage.

Stephens, P. R., Evans, J. R., & Matthews, C. H. (2005). Importance and implementation of Baldrige practices for small businesses. *Quality Management Journal, 12*(3), 21-38.

Stone, P. W., Glied, S. A., McNair, P. D., Matthes, N., Cohen, B., Landers, T. F., & Larson, E. L. (2010). CMS changes in reimbursement for HAIs: Setting a research agenda. *Medical Care, 48*, 433-441.

Suarez, J. G. (1992). *Three experts on quality management: Philip B. Crosby, W. Edwards Deming, Joseph M. Juran* (No. TQLO-PUB-92-02). Total Quality Leadership Office. Arlington VA. Retrieved from http://www.dtic.mil/dtic/tr/fulltext/u2/a256399.pdf

The National Institute of Standards and Technology (NIST). (2011). *2011–2012 Criteria for performance excellence.* Retrieved from http://www.nist.gov/baldrige/publications/upload/2011_2012_Business_Nonprofit_Criteria.pdf

The National Institute of Standards and Technology. (2008). *Baldrige national quality program. The Malcolm Baldrige National Quality Improvement Act of 1987-Public Law 100-107.* Retrieved from http://www.quality.nist.gov/Improvement_Act.html

The National Institute of Standards and Technology. (2010). *Baldrige national quality program. Healthcare criteria for performance excellence.* Retrieved from www.baldrige.nist.gov\

Toussaint, J. (2009). Writing the new playbook for US health care: Lessons from Wisconsin. *Health Affairs, 28,* 1343-1350.

Tralib, F., & Rahman, Z. (2010). Critical success factors of TQM in service organizations: A proposed model. *Services Marketing Quarterly, 31,* 363-380.

Trisolini, M. G., Pope, G. C., Mitchell, J. B., & Greenwald, L. M. (2011). *Pay-for-performance in health care: Methods and approaches.* Triangle Park, NC: RTI Press.

U.S. Department of Health and Human Services. (2011). *Report to Congress: National strategy for quality improvement in health care.* U.S. Department of Health and Human Services. Retrieved from http://www.healthcare.gov/law/resources/reports/quality03212011a.html#tni

U.S. Department of Health and Human Services. (2012). *Report to Congress. Medicare-medicaid.* U.S. Department of Health and Human Services. Retrieved from http://www.cms.gov/Medicare-Medicaid-Coordination/Medicare-and-Medicaid-Coordination/Medicare-Medicaid-Coordination-Office/Downloads/MMCO_2012_RTC_v2.pdf

VanLare, J. M., Moody-Williams, J., & Conway, P. H. (2012). Value-based purchasing for hospitals. *Health Affairs, 31*(1), 249-249.

Wachter, R. M. (2004). The end of the beginning: Patient safety five years after 'To Err Is Human'. *Health Affairs,* 23534-23545. doi:10.1377/hlthaffw4.526

Wachter, R. M. (2010). Patient safety at ten: Unmistakable progress, troubling gaps. *Health Affairs, 29,* 165-173.

Werner, R. M., & McNutt, R. (2009). A new strategy to improve quality. *JAMA: The Journal of the American Medical Association, 301,* 1375-1377.

Werner, R. M., Bradlow, E. T., & Asch, D. A. (2008). Does hospital performance on process measures directly measure high quality care or is it a marker of unmeasured care? *Health Services Research, 43,* 1464-1484.

Werner, R. M., Kolstad, J. T., Stuart, E. A., & Polsky, D. (2011). The effect of pay-for-performance in hospitals: Lessons for quality improvement. *Health Affairs, 30,* 690-698. Retrieved from http://search.proquest.com.library.capella.edu/docview/864026277?accountid=27965

Why not the best? (2011). *Commonwealth fund. Results from the national scorecard on the U.S. health system performance, 2011.* Retrieved from http://www.commonwealthfund.org/Publications/Fund-Reports/2011/Oct/Why-Not-the-Best-2011.aspx?page=all

Wilding, C., & Whiteford, G. (2005). Phenomenological research: An exploration of conceptual, theoretical, and practical issues. *OTJR: Occupation, Participation, and Health, 25*(3), 98-101.

Williams, T. A. (2004). Do you believe in Baldrige? *Quality, 43*(5), 6-6.

Wilson, D. D., & Collier, D. A. (2000). An empirical investigation of the Malcolm Baldrige national quality award causal model. *Decision Sciences, 31,* 361-383.

Yaacob, Z. (2010). Quality management as an effective strategy of cost savings. *African Journal of Aquatic Business Management, 4,* 1844-1855.

Yeung, A. L., Cheng, T., & Kee-hung, L. (2006). An operational and institutional perspective on Total Quality Management. *Production and Operations Management, 15*(1), 156-170.

Yin, R. K. (2009). *Case study research. Design and methods* (4th ed.) Thousand Oaks, CA: Sage.

Yin, R. K. (2003). *Case study research: Design and methods* (3rd ed.). Thousand Oaks, CA: Sage.

Young, N. D. (2002). *The effects of the Malcolm Baldrige national quality award* criteria on the learning systems of selected educational institutions: A study of six state Baldrige-based quality award program winners. (Doctoral dissertation). Retrieved from ProQuest Dissertation and Theses. (UMI 3041621)

Yusuf, Y., Gunasekaran, A., & Dan, G. (2007). Implementation of TQM in China and organisation performance: An empirical investigation. *Total Quality Management, 18*, 509-530.

APPENDICES

APPENDIX A

STATEMENT OF ORIGINAL WORK

Academic Honesty Policy

Capella University's Academic Honesty Policy (3.01.01) holds learners accountable for the integrity of work they submit, which includes but is not limited to discussion postings, assignments, comprehensive exams, and the dissertation or capstone project.

Established in the Policy are the expectations for original work, rationale for the policy, definition of terms that pertain to academic honesty and original work, and disciplinary consequences of academic dishonesty. Also stated in the Policy is the expectation that learners will follow APA rules for citing another person's ideas or works.

The following standards for original work and definition of *plagiarism* are discussed in the Policy:

Learners are expected to be the sole authors of their work and to acknowledge the authorship of others' work through proper citation and reference. Use of another person's ideas, including another learner's, without proper reference or citation constitutes plagiarism and academic dishonesty and is prohibited conduct. (p. 1)

Plagiarism is one example of academic dishonesty. Plagiarism is presenting someone else's ideas or work as your own. Plagiarism also includes copying verbatim or rephrasing ideas without properly acknowledging the source by author, date, and publication medium. (p. 2)

Capella University's Research Misconduct Policy (3.03.06) holds learners accountable for research integrity. What constitutes research misconduct is discussed in the Policy:

> *Research misconduct includes but is not limited to falsification, fabrication, plagiarism, misappropriation, or other practices that seriously deviate from those that are commonly accepted within the academic community for proposing, conducting, or reviewing research, or in reporting research results. (p. 1)*

Learners failing to abide by these policies are subject to consequences, including but not limited to dismissal or revocation of the degree.

Statement of Original Work and Signature

I have read, understood, and abided by Capella University's Academic Honesty Policy (3.01.01) and Research Misconduct Policy (3.03.06), including the Policy Statements, Rationale, and Definitions.

I attest that this dissertation is my own work. Where I have used the ideas or words of others, I have paraphrased, summarized, or used direct quotes following the guidelines set forth in the APA *Publication Manual*.

Mentor name and school	Dr. Suzanne Richins, School of Business and Technology
Learner signature and date	Nicole B. Dhanraj July 17, 2013

APPENDIX B

INTERVIEW QUESTIONNAIRE

(adapted from NIST, 2013)

Interview RS #:

My research is based on health-care reform-Medicare's value based health care where the idea is to increase quality while lowering costs to produce outcomes as mandated by Medicare, otherwise organizations are at risk for losing some of their reimbursement.

The goal is to develop a guideline with the best business practices that organizations can use to facilitate their success as they transition from a fee for service to a fee for performance.

Leadership

Question 1: How would you define quality?
Question 2: What does value based care mean to you?
Question 3: What is the best manner to transform a culture to one of value-based health care?
Question 4: How do you prevent becoming overwhelmed?
Question 5: How do you get "buy in" from staff

especially if they think they are doing a good job?
Question 6: What do you think are the best
mechanisms to share the vision of Value based care?
Question 7: What type of leadership behavior is
ideal?

Customer Focus and Market Focus

Question 8: What is the best way to improve the
value of care for patients?
Question 9: How should leadership respond to the
customer's demands?
Question 10: How much does the "voice of the
customer" affect initiative, processes impact the value
of care?
Question 11: How do you avoid getting overwhelmed
by customer expectations?
Question 12: Can organizations focus on both the
patient and the bottom line?

Workforce Focus

Question 13: What should be the frequency of
training for "front line" employees need to increase the
value of care provided?
Question 14: How should employees be developed to
increase efficiency?
Question 15: What about time and resources?
Question 16: How best is it to introduce change
without causing frustration from staff?
Question 17: How should you incentivize employees
to maintain a culture based on value rather than
volume and payment?

Strategy and Development

Question 18: In your experience, what are some key cost-effective management strategies?

Question 19: How does emphasizing the value of care rather than focusing on volume and payment affect the short and long-term goals of the organization?

Question 20: What are key strategies used to improve efficiency?

Question 21: How do you avoid becoming over ambitious?

Question 22: How do monitor the amount of resources used?

Operation Focus

Question 23: What are the processes used to shift the focus to value in care as opposed to increasing volume?

Question 24: What are some destructive effects of value-based health care on operations?

Question 25: What do you consider to be operation efficiency?

Measurement and Analysis

Question 26: How important is integrating data to improving efficiency?

Question 27: What is the best way to use performance findings to change or improve work processes for better efficiency?

Question 28: How do you devote resources to this venture?

Results

Question 29: What key data (e.g., A/R, patient satisfaction, length of stay) are necessary to set performance targets?

Question 30: How often should performance results be reviewed?

Question 31: How should success in Medicare's value-based health care be measured?

Question 32: How are unintended consequences of moving to fee for performance avoided?

Question 33: Is there any area that you think is important to address as organizations try to find the balance between achieving high quality while lowering costs and remaining financially viable?

INDEX

CURRICULUM VITAE

Nicole Dhanraj

LinkedIn: https://www.linkedin.com/in/nicoledhanraj

Teaching Philosophy

It is my belief that through education, a student receives foundational skills such as writing, collecting, and organizing research, self-management, and creativity, all necessary to shape their future and build a successful and fulfilled life. Within the educational setting, students should be continually encouraged to apply knowledge learned to solve problems related to those they will encounter outside of the classroom setting.

The US Army's core values of duty, integrity and selfless service promoted my development as a determined leader and educator with the coping skills to dig deep and muster the strength to achieve goals regardless of adversity faced. As a military veteran deployed to various duty stations around the world, I had the opportunity to engage with various cultures, languages, and practices. This worldly involvement paired with my experience as a multidisciplinary instructor, and international speaker supports my ability to integrate diversity and subject matter to achieve learning outcomes.

I enjoy working with diverse groups as I believe it is through varied opinions that we learn to broaden our minds and understand differences. It is crucial that each student is recognized for his or her strengths and contributions and given credibility within the course room setting. I believe that students thrive in a positive atmosphere. I endorse such an environment through continuous clear feedback. I promote a flexible and open classroom environment that allows students to think and collaborate independently or as a team which fosters self-determination and confidence in their competence.

My background in the health sector allows me to spot problems and that may affect student performance and as such help them seek the necessary help to avoid unnecessary failure. As a teacher, I recognize the individuality of each student and am drawn to the opportunity to fuel their desire to succeed and contribute to their intellectual growth. I am respectful of diversity and always strive to foster an environment where I can mentor the scholarly development of each student especially through my experience as an author and academic researcher.

As an experienced traditional and online student, I have first-hand knowledge of what is required to adapt to each environment and to produce competent and knowledgeable students, with renewed energy to embrace their future classes. My goal as an educator is to promote active involvement from students by creating rich content that is challenging and promotes critical thinking and creativity in application of content. Through such active involvement, I monitor students' digestion of the subject.

Being transparent, approachable, and sensitive to student's needs creates a sense of willingness to engage in feedback that I can use to improve class participation and strengthen my teaching strategies for future classes.

Education

Capella University, Minneapolis, MN
- Doctor of Philosophy, Organizational Management 2013
- *Dissertation – Exploratory Case Study of the Best Business Practices in Medicare's Value-based Health Care System*

Troy University, Troy, AL
- Master of Science, Magna Cum Laude, 2004
- Major: International Relations

St. Martin's University, Lacey, WA
- Bachelor of Science 2002
- Major: Psychology
- Minor: History

Training & Certifications

Association of Medical Imaging Management, MA
- Certified Radiology Administrator, 2016

Education Consulting and Teaching Experience

Adjunct Professor
University of Maryland University College
Adelphi, MD
2017 – present

- Teach in a hybrid format the strategic role of human resource management.
- The objective is to provide students the knowledge that applies to human behavior, labor relations, and current laws and regulations to a working environment.

- Topics include employment laws and regulations, diversity in a global economy, total rewards management, and training and development for organizational success.

Peer Reviewer
Association of Medical Imaging Management,
Sudbury, MA
2016 – Present

- Responsible for peer reviewing clinical presentations comprising various radiology topics, for example, coding, MRI, safety, management.
- Evaluate the outline to ensure relevance, accuracy, presence of clear objectives, and sufficient time allotted for content.
- Review the faculty's education and/or experience to determine if qualified to deliver subject/content.

Adjunct Professor (Online)
PIMA Community College
Tucson, AZ
2014 – 2017

- Designed and developed course curriculum for health education class.
- Served as an online adjunct as part of the BS program for radiology and respiratory.
- Provided instruction and conduct classes in accordance with the philosophy of the College and within the course of study defined by the department.
- Met all assigned classes with adequate preparation.
- Evaluated student performance and conduct fair evaluations applied equally to all students.
- Attended scheduled meetings called by authorized personnel.

Education Content Reviewer / Medical Advisor
Radiology Info
Oak Brook, IL
2015 - Present

- Responsible for peer reviewing online clinical publications within the radiology field.
- Evaluate the online content to ensure accuracy and up-to-date effective information.
- Provide and edit content related to radiology procedures to be easily understood by members of the public.

Education Content Reviewer
Elsevier
Maryland Heights, MS
2015 - Present

- Responsible for evaluating an organization's compliance with the journal's standards for excellence.
- Responsible for peer reviewing chapters to validate research in the support of submitted work.
- Evaluate the integrity of work submitted to identify invalid research.
- Provide specific comments to authors for suggestions, revisions, and other ways to improve the strength of reviewed manuscripts.

Subject Matter Expert/Contractor
Western Governors University
Salt Lake City, UT
2015 - 2017

- Apply subject matter expertise and insight for the development of the Test Specifications Workshop for Bachelor's and Master's Degree Courses.
- Advise on assessment practices through the development of evidence statements to effectively measure student's competencies.

- Collaborate and network with other subject matter experts and provide robust feedback to ensure that required competencies are relevant to the success of the graduate.

Lecture Circuit Speaker
Medical Technology Management Institute
Menomonee Fall, WI
2014 - Present

- Develop and prepare course materials for various computed tomography classes such as protocol development, radiation safety, image optimization, and case studies.
- Prepare radiology curricula to include computed tomography incorporating the content specifications mandated by the American Registry of radiologic technologists.
- Ensure the anticipated outcomes of the courses were met, following the rubric of MTMI and Herzing University.
- Lectures include:
    CT Registry Review
    CT Protocol Development: Getting it Right
    CT Training Course for Technologists

Owner/Academic Coach Volunteer
HND Online Writing Services
Puyallup, WA
2013 - 2016

- Tailor academic coaching services in improving writing skills through planning, organizing and drafting papers.
- Provide professional, academic, and creative writing needs and assisted in areas in need of improvement.
- Perform duties as a coach in areas of expertise to include academic essays, theses, dissertations, newsletters, and business proposals.

Articles, Presentations, and Research

Dhanraj, N. (2017). The Flipped Classroom Model: Strategies & Tools for Successful Teaching and Student Engagement Experiences in Radiology Schools. Presented as a poster presentation at RadiologyAsia 2017.

Dhanraj, N. (2017). Think Global Radiology. CMRT, October.

Dhanraj, N. (2017). Professional Adrenaline. ASRT Scanner, 49 (5).

Dhanraj, N. (2017). Mentoring Benefits. ISRRT Newsletter, April.

Dhanraj, N., Mazal, J. (2016). Neglected Tropical Diseases in the Americas: The Role of Radiology has been accepted. Presented as a poster presentation at RadiologyAsia 2017.

Presented at the 2016 Annual Meeting of Radiological Society of North America.

Dhanraj, N.& Mazal, J. (2016). "Zika Virus: Implications for Medical Imaging Professionals". Radiologic Technology, 87(6)

Dhanraj, N. (2016). "The Big and Small Issues of the Disproportionate Patient: Technical and Safety Challenges in Radiology." Presented at the 74th Annual General Conference, June 2016 Halifax, Nova Scotia, Canada.

Dhanraj, N., & Rzemyk, T. (2016) Unexploded Ordnances: Approaches to Mitigate Additional Post (Natural) Disaster Risk and Support Environmental Sustainability and Community Reconstruction." To be presented at the University of Massachusetts-Boston, November 2018, International Conference: Disaster Risk Reduction, Response and Sustainable Reconstruction: Capacity Building for Equitable Planning and Development.

Dhanraj, N., & Rzemyk, T. (2016). Scholarly Academic Paper & International Presentation: "The Balancing Act of Economic Growth and Environment Preservation: A Case Study of Guam". Presented at the International Tomorrow's People Organization's Sustainable

Development Conference: Green technology, Renewable Energy and Environmental Protection, July 2016 Kuching, Malaysia.

Dhanraj, N., Johnson-Lutz, H., & Rzemyk, T. (2015) "Women and Economic Development in Post Conflict Afghanistan: Learning from Other Muslim Nations.". Presented at University of Massachusetts-Boston, July 2015, International Conference: Rebuilding Sustainable Communities in Afghanistan - The Way Forward July 2015.

Presented at Tomorrow People Organization's 7th Annual Women's Leadership and Empowerment Conference, March 2016, Bangkok, Thailand. Presented at Tomorrow People Organization 7th Annual Women's Leadership and Empowerment Conference, March 2016, Bangkok, Thailand.

Dhanraj, N. B. (2013). An exploratory case study of the business practices for success in Medicare's value-based health care program (Doctoral dissertation, CAPELLA UNIVERSITY. Presented at the Tomorrow People Organization's Public Health Conference July 2016, Kuching, Malaysia.

Professional Positions

Guam Memorial Hospital
Tamuning, GU
2015-present
Chief of Radiology Services

- Monitors department operations through interactions with Radiologist, supervisory personnel, and department personnel. Improved department patient flow by 70% in two years.

- Interviews, appoints, and terminated employees, maintains individual personnel files, discusses grievances with employees.

- Collaboratively formulates departmental targets and goals with Chairman of Radiology and Administrator of Professional Support Services.
- Adopts prudent financial practices such as inventory control, cost ratio's, and cost benefit analysis to maintain efficient operations within the department.
- Prepares budgets for presentation to Administration and Local Legislature.
- Provides ongoing reassessment of departmental cost effectiveness and productivity. Reduced unnecessary expenses by 30% through various cost control measures.
- Develops annual and long-range capital equipment acquisition and replacement plan. Presented business plan to Governor as part of a hospital improvement project. Procured $2M in equipment in two years.
- Processes all Department requisitions for supplies and equipment.
- Maintains a Quality Assurance and Quality Control Program for the department of Radiology. Significant overall improvement for previous Medicare and Joint Commission citations.
- Advises employees on all new personnel policies and changes which affect the Department.
- Hold regular scheduled monthly meetings with staff. Increased staff communication and awareness of operations.
- Responsible for ensuring accurate coding and reporting. Reduced coding errors by 75%.
- Manage, monitor and maintain PACS, RIS, Imaging systems and applications to ensure maximum uptime. IT errors within the department improved 90%.
- Reviews dosimetry reports for staff as well as patient dose reports for CT.
- Functions as a resource person for staff members and assists in necessary education of individual members of the staff and hospital staff.
- Evaluates and provides solutions to risk management and administration of department safety issues.

- Restarted hospital mammography program that was dormant for 5 years.
- Work with multiple vendors to improve existing services as well as procure new equipment/supplies.
- Coordinates with outside facilities to facilitate care when department services unavailable.
- Solicite feedback from others department such as the Operating Room, Special Services, and Nursing to incorporate improvement opportunities into goal setting.
- Maintain compliance to regulatory and local standards and policies.
- Function as the superuser for the RIS and HIS systems.
- Provide a resource for co-workers in other areas on inpatient and outpatient charge document review, and on coding.

Technical operations Director;
Chief MR/CT Technologist
Sound Medical Imaging
Puyallup, WA
2005 – 2010

- Troubleshot all clinical issues, including PACS and RIS issues; Supported the reduction of expensive service calls by 25%.
- Developed and maintained relationships with referring providers and prospective groups. Identified new groups and providers, increasing referrals by 30%, and adding new services to the practice.
- Worked with senior management to use business intelligence to assess competitors and developed subsequent business plans, resulting in a 40% increase in patient volume.
- Ensured compliance to standards through ongoing measurement and monitoring regularly with developmental action plans to improve performance.

- Managed vendor relationships to ensure quality service, including timeliness and cost effectiveness of vendor products and services.
- Established and maintained collaborative relationships with external partners.
- Analyzed staff capabilities and established priorities for advancement opportunities within the organization.
- Frequently communicated with Radiologists to maintain a productive working relationship.

MR / CT / Interventional Technologist / Radiology Technologist
Diagnostic imaging (Contractor)
Western WA
2002 - Present

- Licensed Radiologic Technologist, experienced in general radiology, CT Scan, MRI Scan and Interventional Radiology within multiple healthcare settings of medical imaging.
- Promoted cost effective strategies through continuous elevation of processes for improvement resulting in improved patient satisfaction and enhanced efficiencies of operational workflow.
- Responsible for the training of new technologists, delivering safety, technical, and customer service presentations.

Entrepreneurial Experience

Owner/Operations Director
HND Enterprise
Puyallup, WA
2005 - 2013

- Controlled all aspects of business development projects to maximize resources, revenue and productivity through strategic development and critical

thinking, consistently enhancing the business for eight consecutive years.
- Facilitated business growth opportunities though competitive market analysis, product development and creative marketing strategies, increasing sales by 30%
- Trained and provided guidance to employees, with a significant emphasis on customer service, resulting in a 95% customer satisfaction rating.
- Consistently maintained a high standard of performance with strong attention to detail, consequently building a large and loyal customer base.

Military Service

Sergeant / CT/Radiology Technologist
US Army Medical Centers (Secret Clearance.
(Academic & Training) WA & Germany)
2000 – 2003

- Trained 50 diagnostic technologists at the hospital and ten outlying clinics to become CT proficient, in Germany and Kosovo.
- Designed, wrote, and implemented a protocol manual for the department and ten outlying clinics, resulting in consistent imaging techniques across all worksites.
- Managed assets valued at more than $1.75M.
- Army Commendation Medal; Army Achievement Medal (3rd Award); National Defense Medal; Army Service Ribbon; Army Lapel Button, Honorable Discharge.

Volunteer Experience

- **SCORE, 2015** Share expertise and mentor small business owners to meet their goals and achieve success in their own business both face to face and online. Assist in providing education and training to soldiers as part of the Department of Defense's Transition Assistance Program in the Boots to

Business Program.
- **Teaching Practice Seminar, 2012**. Examined the practice fundamentals necessary for a teaching career as well as explored the fundamentals of human development for success in the classroom.
- **Club Z Tutoring**, **2004-2006,** Puyallup, WA, Prepared and developed creative lesson plans for high school and college students that enabled their success.
- **Radiology Continuing Education Workshop**, **2000**, Madigan Army Medical Center. Coordinated radiologic classes for employees to ensure understanding of techniques and delivery of quality imaging work.
- **Military In-service Training Workshops, 2000**, Madigan Army Medical Center, Wurzburg Army Medical Center, 2002-2003. Liaised with department supervisors and military leadership to teach didactic clinical and military classes to soldiers within the department as well as outlying clinics. Appointed as a subject matter expert in Computed Tomography as well as various military subjects and was responsible for providing quarterly training.
- **Student Mentorship Program for Radiology Students**, **2000**, Army Medical Department, San Antonio, TX. Subject matter expert to mentor failing students, contributed to 100% graduation rate.
- **HND Online Writing Service, 2014-2016:** Provide guidance and mentorship as an academic coach for undergraduate and graduate students specifically with research organization, and editing.
- **Diva Docs, 2014-2017,** Weekly contributor on an online internet radio show designed to motivate and empower doctoral learners. Responsible for interviewing and commentating with guests regarding their experiences that contributed to their success.
- **PhD Sisters Group, 2012 – present.** Serve as a peer mentor and advisor for doctoral learners. Provide direct guidance for students to support their academic success. Subject matter expert on research design, content organization, and data analysis.

- **RAD-AID, 2016-present.** Serve as an onsite volunteer for local projects as needed as well as resource for the online learning management center. Responsible for setting up accounts for end users, creating and uploading content, troubleshooting website issues and recruiting authors as well as other volunteers.
- **Joint Women's Leadership, Guam, 2016-present.** Serve as secretary in coordinating and planning annual women's leadership event in conjunction with the US Military. Was guest speaker at 2017 leadership symposium.

Professional Affiliations

- American College of Healthcare Executives
- Washington State Healthcare Executives
- The Association for Medical Imaging Management
- Institute for Healthcare Improvement
- Dissertation Coaches
- Healthcare Financial Management Association

Platforms

Blackboard, WebCT, LEO, Moodle

Subject Matter Expert Areas

- Curriculum Development
- Learner-Centered Instructional Strategies
- Flipped Classrooms
- Distance Education
- Health Education
- Healthcare Leadership & Healthcare Operations
- Computed Tomography
- Magnetic Resonance Imaging

- Radiology Technology
- Regulatory Compliance
- Conflict Management
- Development
- Entrepreneurship
- Human Resources Management
- International Business & International Relations
- Management & Project Management
- Management and Organizational Theory
- Microfinance
- Organizational Behavior
- Organizational Communication
- Organizational Leadership
- Organizational Transformation and development
- Risk Management
- Sustainability

Personal Attributes and Qualifications

- ***Communication skills***. Highly organized individual skilled at providing clear and effective expectations and guidance when interacting with customers, team members or leadership. Experienced in technical, business, and academic writing using APA and MLA formats. Experienced lecturer, circuit speaker. Multilingual.

- ***Performer***. Known for a commitment to excellence, a talent for creative solutions, and a capacity to motivate and instill confidence in the course room and in practitioner work. Solid 15 years of mentoring and teaching experience with consistent excellent results.
- ***Analytical and Metacognitive.*** Led multiple projects through evaluation, strategy development, problem solving, creativity, and collective educated decision-making to achieve projected time and budget goals. Used business analytics and statistics to critically

understand market conditions. Knowledge of statistical software such as Nvivo, SPSS and Atlas.ti.

- *Leadership skills.* Capable of executing various leadership styles according to situation or environment. Adept and able to multitask, work on complex projects, and function productively in stressful times. Thorough and attentive to detail; a self-starter who can work independently or as a productive contributor in a team.
- *Reliable.* Can always be counted on, and trusted to get any task done right and efficiently. Adept and able to multitask, work on complex projects, and function productively in stressful times.
- *Flexible.* Accepts change, capable of rapidly adapting to change within industry or through management directional changes.
- *Creative.* Able to assess, and synthesize information to shape business plans and goals to consistently maintain the competitive advantage and stay abreast with technology and literature within the field.
- *Passion.* Possess an ardent desire consistently perform duties optimally and grow professionally. Known for a commitment to excellence, and a talent for creative solutions.

ABOUT THE AUTHOR

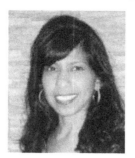

Dr. Nicole B. Dhanraj received her Bachelor's Degree in Psychology from St Martin's University and her Master's in International Relations, graduating magna cum laude from Troy State University. She earned her doctorate with an emphasis in Organizational Management from Capella University. She is considered a subject matter expert on the technical, managerial, and operational aspects of healthcare. Dr. Dhanraj began her career in radiology as a diagnostic imaging and CT technologist in the US Army, and her background also includes clinical work in interventional radiology and MRI.

Dr. Dhanraj is passionate about global radiology and seeks to strengthen the international radiology community through empowering others with her knowledge. She is a recent recipient of the 2016 ASRT Foundation International Speaker Exchange Award in Canada and the 2016 ASRT Foundation Community Outreach Fellow for Cape Verde. She is a volunteer with RAD-AID, serves as an ambassador with the World Radiography Educational Trust Foundation (WRETF) and is an active member with the International Society of Radiographers and Radiological Technologists.

She co-authored the article, *Zika Virus: Implications for Medical Imaging Professionals*, published in the July/August 2016 issue of *Radiologic Technology*. She is dedicated to issues such poverty, entrepreneurship, environment, and women affairs and has presented at international conferences on topics related to these issues. When she is not saving the world one x-ray at a time, she works as a researcher, an educator, and as the Director of Radiology at Guam Memorial Hospital, in Guam.

CONTACT THE AUTHOR

You may contact the author with questions, comments, or continuing research inquiries at:

nicoledhanrajbooks@gmail.com

ABOUT THE BOOK

This book is a must read for health-care organization leaders. This research is of significance for the health-care organizations looking for a fresh approach to use resources appropriately to reduce waste, increase value of services, deliver the quality of health care the system as intended, and enable health care organization leaders to maintain their financially profitable status. This study supports the need for evidence-based business strategies that facilitates success in participating organizations of Medicare's value-based program and a redefinition of financial sustainability in health care that emphasizes value.

Within the health-care industry, numerous quality improvement strategies exist to promote a more efficient and effective system. Despite such strategies, the health-care system is yet to experience sustained quality improvement. Value-based health care is a pecuniary strategy established by the Center of Medicare and Medicaid Services to achieve sustained improvement, both in the delivery of care and in clinical outcomes.

Medicare provides clinical process measures as a guideline for organizations in delivering higher quality with a value-based strategy. This strategy situation may create difficulties for organizations in selecting the most suitable business strategies that maintain a quality-financial balance. Leaders are left to guess at business strategies most optimal for success in the program, as well as for the organization's financial sustainability.

Sustained improvement in the health-care industry can be accelerated when leaders are knowledgeable on appropriate strategies important to increasing the value and quality of care, while reducing waste. This exploratory qualitative study used the Malcolm Baldrige Criteria for Performance Excellence as a quality improvement tool for exploring the business strategies can promote clinical and financial success for organizations participating in Medicare's value-based program.

Made in the USA
Las Vegas, NV
01 November 2023

80074711R00164